Wissenschaftliche Beiträge
zur Medizinelektronik

Band 10

T0140859

Wissenschaftliche Beiträge zur Medizinelektronik

Band 10

Herausgegeben von
Prof. Dr. Wolfgang Krautschneider

Jan Claudio Loitz

Novel Methods in Electrical Stimulation with Surface Electrodes

Logos Verlag Berlin

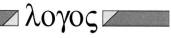

Wissenschaftliche Beiträge zur Medizinelektronik

Herausgegeben von
Prof. Dr. Wolfgang Krautschneider

Technische Universität Hamburg-Harburg
Institut für Nano- und Medizinelektronik
Eißendorfer Str. 38
D-21073 Hamburg

Bibliografische Information der Deutschen Nationalbibliothek

Die Deutsche Nationalbibliothek verzeichnet diese Publikation in der
Deutschen Nationalbibliografie; detaillierte bibliografische Daten sind
im Internet über http://dnb.d-nb.de abrufbar.

ISBN 978-3-8325-4885-8
ISSN 2190-3905

Logos Verlag Berlin GmbH
Comeniushof, Gubener Str. 47,
10243 Berlin
Tel.: +49 (0)30 / 42 85 10 90
Fax: +49 (0)30 / 42 85 10 92
http://www.logos-verlag.de

Novel Methods in Electrical Stimulation with Surface Electrodes

Vom Promotionsausschuss der
Technischen Universität Hamburg
zur Erlangung des akademischen Grades
Doktor-Ingenieur (Dr.-Ing.)

genehmigte Dissertation

von
Jan Claudio Loitz

aus
Bad Oldesloe, Deutschland

2019

1. Gutachter: Prof. Dr.-Ing. Wolfgang H. Krautschneider
2. Gutachter: Prof. Dr. habil. Michael M. Morlock

Tag der mündlichen Prüfung: 28.11.2018

Danksagung

An erster Stelle gilt mein Dank meinem Doktorvater Herr Prof. Wolfgang Krautschneider für seine wissenschaftliche und methodische Unterstützung während der gesamten Bearbeitungsphase. Prof. Dr. Michael Morlock danke ich für die Zweitbegutachtung meiner Arbeit und Prof. Dr. Manfred Kasper für die Übernahme des Prüfungsvorsitzes. Außerdem bedanke ich mich bei Dr. Dietmar Schröder für seine stets offene Tür und viele zielführende und anregende Diskussionen. Ein großer Dank geht an Ute Schmitd und alle Institutsmitarbeiter, die mich bei der Bearbeitung mit Ihrer anhaltenden Hilfestellung begleitet haben.

Aljoscha Reinert danke ich für die zahlreichen fachlichen Gespräche, die mich immer wieder neue Aspekte und Ansätze entdecken ließen, besonders während der Mittagspause.

Ein großer Dank gilt meinen Eltern, die mich immer mit allen Mitteln unterstützt haben und dessen Erziehung ich meine große Neugier zu verdanken habe. Freunden und Familie danke ich für Ihre unermüdliche Stärkung und Motivation.

Besonders danken möchte ich meiner Frau Regina Loitz dafür, dass sie mir immer mit Rat und Tat zur Seite steht, sie unendlich geduldig mit mir ist und dafür, dass sie mich immer wieder anspornt und mich ermutigt nie aufzugeben.

Abstract

Electrical stimulation is a versatile tool used for rehabilitation of patients suffering from central and peripheral nerve lesions and many other medical interventions. Novel methods to improve the application of electrical stimulation with surface electrodes, especially for the treatment of stroke survivors with an upper limb hemiparesis, are derived and presented.

For this purpose a simulation environment is created which can be used to model the response of motor neurons to externally applied stimuli. Insights regarding efficient and indulgent stimulation pulses as well as factors determining optimal stimulation electrode designs are described and discussed.

Difficulties during electrode placement, non-intuitive control methods and an early onset of muscular fatigue often limit the success of electrical stimulation for the treatment of stroke survivors. Therefore, measurements with people living with the consequences of a cerebrovascular accident are performed in cooperation with physicians, leading to concepts for intuitive and effective use of electrical stimulation.

Systems allowing the use of array electrodes, which drastically ease the process of electrode placement and enable precise hand movements, are developed. This also includes an innovative method for rapid prototyping of array electrodes. Intuitive control and compensation of muscular fatigue is achieved by integrating mechanical and myoelectric sensors wirelessly in the developed systems, constituting a distinct improvement compared to currently available systems for neurorehabilitation.

The ideas behind these developments include modularity and up-to-date control over mobile devices, resulting in a concept with a high chance of industrial take-up.

Contents

Glossary

Symbols

c_m	Membrane capacitance per unit area [μF/cm^2]	I	Nodal current [A]
C_m	Membrane capacitance [F]	$(K)_i$	Internal potassium concentration [mM]
d	Axon diameter [μm]	$(K)_o$	external potassium concentration [mM]
ϵ_0	Electric field constant [F/m]		
ϵ_r	Relative permittivity	λ	Space constant
F	Faraday's constant [As/mol]	L	Node of Ranvier length [μm]
G_a	Axial internodal conductance [S]	$(Na)_i$	Internal sodium concentration [mM]
g_m	Membrane conductance per unit area [mS/cm^2]	$(Na)_o$	External sodium concentration [mM]
G_m	Membrane conductance [S]	$\bar{P}_K$	Potassium permeability constant [cm/s]
i_K	Potassium current density [μA/cm^2]	$\bar{P}_{Na}$	Sodium permeability constant [cm/s]
i_{Na}	Sodium current density [μA/cm^2]	$\bar{P}_P$	Nonspecific permeability constant [cm/s]
i_L	Leakage current density [μA/cm^2]	ρ	Electric resistivity [Ωm]
i_P	Nonspecific delayed current density [μA/cm^2]	ρ_i	Specific axoplasm resistance [Ωm]

R	Gas constant [kg m^2/s^2 mol K]	V_i	Intracellular potential [mV]
σ	Electric conductivity [S/m]	V_m	Membrane potential [mV]
T	Temperature in Kelvin [K]	V_r	Resting potential [mV]
T_{stim}	Time frame for stimulation pulse [ms]	V_s	Threshold potential [mV]
V	Electric potential [V]	V_{stim}	System response to an arbitrary stimulus [mV]
$V(t)$	System response to a 1 mA, 1µs pulse [mV]	$\vec{x}_{stim}$	Unit less arbitrary stimulus
V_e	Extracellular potential [mV]	Δx	Internodal distance [mm]

Abbreviations

AC/DC	Alternating Current/Cirect Current	**LTI**	Linear Time Invariant
BLE	Bluetooth Low Energy	**MAV**	Motor Axon Volume
DLFS	Distributed Low Frequency Stimulation	**NMES**	Neuromuscular Electrical Stimulation
EEG	Electroencephalography, Electroencephalogram	**PC**	Personal Computer
		PCB	Printed Circuit Board
EMG	Electromyography, Electromyogram	**SCI**	Spinal Cord Injury
FE	Finite Element	**SPI**	Serial Peripheral Interface
FEM	Finite Element Eethod	**TES**	Transcutaneous Electrical Stimulation
FES	Functional Electrical Stimulation	**TENS**	Transcutaneous Electrical Nerve Stimulation
FPCB	Flexible Printed Circuit Board	**USB**	Universal Serial Bus
I/O	Input/Output		

1 Introduction

Interacting with the surrounding and moving objects with two hands is something natural that most people do not think about. A stroke is a traumatic event leaving many survivors with persistent impairments, one of the most frequent is limited control of the hand as the consequence of a hemiparesis [1].

Electrical stimulation with surface electrodes enables the excitation of motor axons with short electrical pulses, thereby causing muscle contractions [2]. For many years this technique has been employed for rehabilitative treatment [3, 4]. If performed in a coordinated manner, electrical stimulation can be used to perform complex movements such as grasping [5, 6, 7, 8, 9]. Individuals suffering from a spinal cord injury (SCI) or stroke can benefit from coordinated electrical stimulation to supplement lost functions [10].

The requirements for systems that intend to support SCI or stroke patients differ greatly. SCI patients are often bound to a wheelchair and have lost the ability to use both arms, whereas a stroke survivor often maintains some mobility and is only impaired on one half of his body. An individual who has lost both hand functions requires a system that generates complete functional movement patterns, e.g. grasping an object and moving it to the mouth. Such tasks are difficult to achieve solely with electrical stimulation, therefore hybrid approaches using mechanical orthesis can be utilized [11]. Mobility and cosmetics are of minor importance in this case. Even implantable systems are an option and were successfully employed with the Freehand System [12](NeuroControl, Cleveland, Ohio, USA).

An individual with chronic stroke uses his healthy hand for everyday tasks. In most cases electrical stimulation is used for rehabilitative purposes [13, 14, 15, 16, 17, 18]. A complete recovery of hand functions is unfortunately often times not possible and survivors have to live with life-long impairments. Here, systems that can offer some support during daily activities could lead to a quality of life increase. Such systems have to be easy to use and mobile, otherwise no acceptance can be expected. Current systems are quite simple and use predefined parameters rather than ones based on sensor feedback. One example of a simple device enabling hand movements during daily activities is the NESS H200 [19](Bioness, Valencia, CA, USA). In the last couple of years the use of array electrodes was proposed as one method to ease the process of correct electrode placement [20, 21].

In this thesis considerations for improvements of electrical stimulation, especially for stroke survivors, will be presented. Therefore, a simulation environment is developed at first to gain a deeper understanding of the underlying mechanisms. Simulations are then used to assess how applications of electrical stimulation can be designed and performed more effectively. In a later stage concepts of systems for electrical stimulation with surface electrodes are presented and discussed. The popularity of smartphones integrated in medical applications is steadily increasing [22]. This development offers many opportunities due to the intuitive interface smartphones offer for the patient. Of course the increasing popularity of medical applications on smartphones also contains several risks regarding safety and data security [23]. In this thesis smartphone controlled stimulation systems will be introduced. The role of the smartphone can vary from a simple remote control to the core of a feedback controlled multi-component system. Experimental studies are performed to gain knowledge about the effect of electrical stimulation on stroke patients and to assess the effectiveness of stimulation parameters and techniques.

Outline

This thesis is structured in the following way: Chapter 2 of this thesis will describe physiological basics and the principle of electrical stimulation. In Chapter 3 the simulation methods used to model electrical stimulation is explained. Considerations regarding efficient electrical stimulation will be discussed in Chapter 4, ranging from properties of single stimulation pulses through electrode geometries and array electrodes. Chapter 5 will introduce systems for electrical stimulation with array electrodes afterwards. Possibilities to trigger and control stimulations with data acquired by sensors are described in Chapter 6. Presentations of the experimental studies that were performed during this project can be found in Chapter 7. Subsequently, this thesis will be completed with a final conclusion in Chapter 8.

2 Background Information and Theory

In this chapter the fundamentals necessary to understand the effects of external electrical stimuli applied to the human body will be described. The first section will explain some physiological basics of the human nervous system. An introduction to electrical stimulation will be presented in the second section.

2.1 Physiology of the Nervous and Musculoskeletal System

The information presented in this section are based on [24, 25, 26, 27, 28] and aim to provide the reader with a general knowledge on physiology of the nervous and musculoskeletal system. The interested reader is encouraged to have a closer look at the mentioned material or similar resources.

2.1.1 The Nervous System

The nervous system allows an organism to interact with its surrounding environment (somatic nervous system) and its entrails (autonomic nervous system). The somatic nervous system is responsible for conscious perception and movements, whereas the autonomic nervous system controls the function of internal organs unconsciously.

The nervous system is also divided anatomically into two parts: The central nervous system (CNS) and the peripheral nervous system (PNS). The brain and spinal cord form the CNS. All other forms of peripheral nerves and nervous tissue are allocated to the PNS.

Two different neural pathways have to be distinguished by their respective function. First, sensory pathways transmitting information from peripheral sensory organs to the

3

Tab. 2.1. Diameter and conduction velocity of motor axons classified after Erlanger and Gasser [26].

Axon type	Diameter [μm]	Conduction velocity [m/s]
Aα	10 - 20 μm	80 - 120 m/s
Aβ	about 10 μm	about 60 m/s
Aγ	about 5 μm	about 30 m/s

CNS, also called afferent pathways of nerves. Second, motoric pathways transmitting commands from the CNS to peripheral muscles or glands, also called efferent pathways or nerves.

2.1.2 The Neuron

The basic element of the nervous system is the neuron. Multiple neurons can form networks to achieve complex tasks. In these networks neurons are connected to one another through synapses. Even though the tasks and sizes of neurons are varying greatly the general structure remains the same. All neurons have a soma which contains the nucleus and other organelles. Dendrites stretch out to other neurons and enable perception of input signals. The axon is the output of the neuron and can forward signals to neurons or muscle fibers.

Figure 2.1 shows a motor neuron. Axons of motor neurons (motor axons) can be up to 100 cm long, building a direct efferent pathway from the spinal cord to a skeletal muscle. Motor neurons receive and process input signals at the spinal cord from other neurons. These input signals can have an excitatory or inhibitory effect on the neuron. An excitation of the motor neuron will cause an output signal that travels along the axon to the target muscle at the periphery. The connection between an axon and a muscle fiber is called neuromuscular junction. Since motor axons can be very long a high conduction velocity is necessary. Axons were classified depending on their conduction velocity. The fast motor axons were called A fibers (Table 2.1). Aα fibers are the fastest and largest motor axons. They innervate peripheral skeletal muscles and cause conscious contractions.

To increase conduction velocity motor axons are partly covered by a myelin sheath, allowing a faster saltatory conduction. This sheath is formed by Schwann cells that

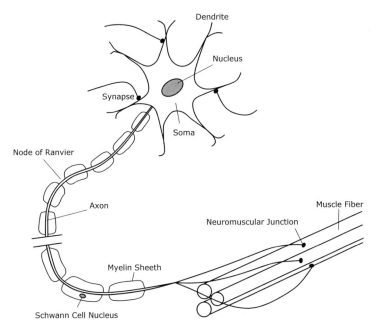

Fig. 2.1. Illustration of a motor neuron. The motor neuron receives signals through
synapses located at the dendrites. Over the motor axon signals are passed to
neuromuscular junctions which activate muscle fibers. One motor neuron can
activate hundreds of muscle fibers. The myelin sheath, separated by nodes of
Ranvier, enables a faster conduction velocity.

wrap around the axon. The myelin sheath builds an isolation of the motor axon that
is interrupted every 1-2 mm by 1-3 µm wide gaps called nodes of Ranvier.

2.1.3 Chemical Synapse

A synapse (Figure 2.2) is the junction between two neurons. Electrical signals from
an axon cause the presynaptic ending to release neurotransmitters which are stored
in synaptic vesicles. The neurotransmitters are released in the synaptic cleft where
receptors at the postsynaptic ending receive them. At the postsynaptic neuron new
electrical signals emerge that can have an excitatory or inhibitory effect on the cell.

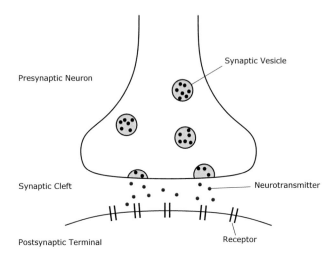

Fig. 2.2. Chemical synapse.

Neuromuscular Junction

A chemical synapse between a neuron and a muscle fiber is called neuromuscular junction. The postsynaptic ending is part of the muscle fiber where the absorption of neurotransmitters results in an electric signal which propagates along the fiber and causes a contraction.

Motor Unit

A motor unit consists of a motor neuron and all muscle fibers it is innervating. All muscle fibers of a motor unit contract together. A large motor unit can include up to 1000 muscle fibers, leading to a coarse contraction strength control of the concerned muscle. Big muscles of the back do typically have large motor units, whereas eye muscles have very small motor units, enabling precise movements.

2.1.4 The Action Potential

The signals traveling along an axon are short electrical pulses called action potentials (AP). They are the foundation for fast and reliable biological communication in the nervous system. Action potentials do not vary in size and shape to encode the strength of a neural signal. Instead the frequency of action potentials determines whether a strong or weak excitation occurs. Strong signals are encoded by a fast frequency of action potentials, whereas weak signals produce low frequencies.

An action potential is a change of the electric potential over the axon membrane. A concentration gradient of charge carriers between the axoplasm (fluid in the inside of the axon) and the extracellular fluid (fluid around the axon) is responsible for the potential difference. The axon membrane has different permeabilities for sodium (Na^+), potassium (K^+) and chloride (Cl^-) ions. The axon membrane has a negative resting potential before any action potentials emerge. The resting potential of a membrane (V_m) can be described by the Goldman equation:

$$V_m = -\frac{RT}{F} \ln \frac{P_K c_{in,K} + P_{Na} c_{in,Na} + P_{Cl} c_{out,Cl}}{P_K c_{out,K} + P_{Na} c_{out,Na} + P_{Cl} c_{in,Cl}} \qquad (2.1)$$

with the gas constant R, the temperature T and the Faraday's constant F. The permeability of the membrane is represented by P_{ion}, $c_{in,ion}$ and $c_{out,ion}$ show the concentration of the respective ions in the inside and outside of the axon. During the resting potential the concentration of K^+ ions is much greater in the inside of the axon compared to the surrounding and the other way around for Na^+ ions. Typical values for resting potentials of axons are between -70 mV and -90 mV.

The permeability of the membrane is controlled by voltage dependent ion channels. An excitatory signal from the soma or an external electrical stimuli can change the membrane potential and thereby the permeability of the membrane for certain ions. The membrane potential has to exceed a threshold potential (e.g. -55 mV) to cause a meaningful change of the membrane permeability which can then result in the emergence of an action potential.

Increasing the membrane potential over the threshold causes Na^+ channels to open, leading to a fast influx of Na^+ ions into the axon. This leads to an depolarization of the membrane potential until a value of about +20 mV is reached. After a short period Na^+ channels will close again and K^+ channels open, resulting in large quantities of K^+ ions leaving the axon. This causes a repolarization of the membrane potential. The fast outflow of K^+ ions leads to a potential more negative than the resulting potential (Hyperpolarization). An active mechanism called Na^+/K^+ATPase supports the restoration and maintenance of the resting potential. Figure 2.3 shows an action potential and the membrane permeability for Na^+ and K^+ ions.

After the start of an action potential a time interval called refractory period determines the time when the next action potential can be triggered. The absolute refractory period lasts until the onset of the hyperpolarization. At this point Na^+ channels are again accessible to stimuli. After the onset of the hyperpolarization until the resting potential is reached an action potential can be triggered but requires a stronger stimuli to reach the threshold potential, this period is called relative refractory period. The absolute refractory period determines the maximum frequency of action potential that can occur. A refractory period of 2 ms would result in a possible frequency of 500 Hz. However, normal signal transfer in the nervous system does not exceed frequencies of 200 Hz.

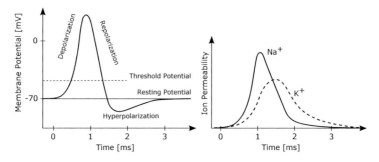

Fig. 2.3. Action potential and membrane permeability.

Action Potential Propagation

An action potential causes a local increase of positive charge carriers in the axon. The surplus of positive charge carriers compared to the neighboring regions cause an internal current flowing from the location of the action potential origin to the not excited parts of the axon. The same happens outside of the axon in the opposite direction. These local currents change the membrane potential along the axon which elicits new action potentials. Thus, causing a propagation of the original action potential (Figure 2.4 (a)).

A myelin sheath forms an insulation between the axon and the extracellular fluid, thereby only eliciting action potentials at the nodes of Ranvier (Figure 2.4 (b)). This so called saltatory conduction results in a greatly increased conduction velocity.
Action potentials also appear at muscle fibers and are caused by neuromuscular junc-

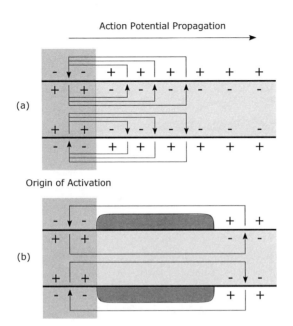

Fig. 2.4. Propagation of an action potential. (a) unmyelinated axon. (b) saltatory conduction of a myelinated axon.

tions. A muscle fiber behaves like non myelinated axons and the action potentials propagate in both directions away from the neuromuscular junction, causing the muscle to contract.

2.1.5 Measuring Muscle Activity

Action potentials at muscle fibers caused by neuromuscular junctions behave like non myelinated axons. The action potentials propagate in both directions away from the neuromuscular junction and cause the muscle to contract. Since one motor axon can activate a large amount of muscle fibers the electric activity during a muscle contraction is considerably greater compared to the electric activity of a nerve bundle. Therefore, the electric activity during a muscle contraction can be measured easily with surface electrodes. This technique is called electromyography (EMG) and the measured signal a electromyogram (EMG).

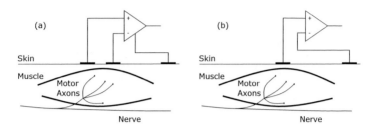

Fig. 2.5. Bipolar (a) and monopolar (b) recording of muscle activity.

The most common electrode configurations to measure muscle activity are monopolar and bipolar recordings [29]. Monololar recordings are performed with one measurement electrode over the muscle belly and a reference electrode placed further away, in the best case over electrically quiet tissue like bones or tendons (Figure 2.5 (b)). Monopolar recordings may include a large amount of noise.

Bipolar recordings use two measurement electrodes (Figure 2.5 (a)). This way the common noise measured by both electrodes can be canceled out, resulting in a higher signal quality.

2.2 Electrical Stimulation of Neural Tissue

In this section electrical stimulation as a rehabilitation technique will be introduced. The here presented information are mainly based on [5] and [2].

The stimulation of neural tissue by electrical means has been a valuable tool for rehabilitation recovery over the last decades. Electrical stimulation can help to increase muscle strength after injuries or even to prevent or reduce muscle atrophy for patients with a spinal cord injury (SCI). Electrical stimulation can help treating pain. Furthermore, muscle contractions caused by electrical stimuli can be used to perform complex movements like grasping or walking to help people suffering from a SCI or stroke.

In the field of electrical stimulation a lot of terms and acronyms are used which should be clarified for the reader at this point. The stimulation of motor axons with the desire to cause muscle contractions can be called 'electrical stimulation' (ES) or 'neuromuscular electrical stimulation' (NMES). As soon as the elicited movement shall be used to achieve functional tasks or to supplement lost functions the term 'functional electrical stimulation' (FES) is used. Applying electrical stimulation pulses to reduce pain is a technique referred to as 'transcutaneous electrical nerve stimulation' (TENS). TENS should not be confused with 'transcutaneous electrical stimulation' (TES) which just describes that stimulation pulses are applied via transcutaneously (on the surface of the skin) placed electrodes. TES does not indicate the purpose of the stimulation.

2.2.1 Principle

During electrical stimulation short pulses from a stimulation device are delivered to a patient through electrodes. These electrodes can be implanted or placed on the skin. At least two electrodes are used during electrical stimulation. The stimulation current causes an ion flow in the tissue. Positive charge carriers accumulate beneath the cathode, negative charge carriers beneath the anode. The local accumulation of positive ions close to the cathode depolarizes the membrane potential of motor axons which can result in the generation of action potentials, if the threshold potential is overcome. The activation of many motor axons can result in a visible and strong muscle contraction. Since activation of motor neurons happens predominantly beneath the cathode it is often called active electrode. The anode on the other hand is often referred to as indifferent electrode. Figure 2.6 illustrates the basic principle of electrical stimulation with surface electrodes.

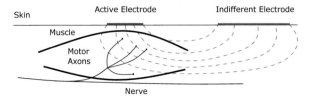

Fig. 2.6. Electrical stimulation with surface electrodes. Active and indifferent electrodes are placed on the skin. Stimulation current can flow from one electrode to the other, passing motor axons that innervate the target muscle.

2.2.2 Stimulation Parameters

Electrical stimulation is typically performed with stimulation pulses that have a rectangular biphasic shape (Figure 2.7). After the stimulation pulse a second pulse with the opposite polarity is applied to reverse the displacement of charge carriers. Hereby, a long lasting accumulation of unilateral polarized charge carriers is avoided which might otherwise lead to cauterizations beneath the electrodes.

The reverse pulse is not supposed to have an impact on the actual stimulation, therefore an interphase of typically $100\,\mu s$ is often added between both pulses. The stimulation intensity is determined by the frequency of the stimulation pulses, the amplitude as well as the pulse width.

Frequency

The number of stimulation pulses per second delivered by the stimulation device to the electrodes is the stimulation frequency. Each stimulation pulse will trigger a cascade of action potentials, resulting in a short muscle twitch. To produce a smooth (tetanic) contraction respectively movement a certain frequency is necessary. With increasing frequency single twitches elicited by individual stimulation pulses add up, first to a incomplete tetanus followed by a complete tetanus (Figure 2.8). The frequencies used for electrical stimulation with tetanic contractions are between 20 and $50\,\mathrm{Hz}$.

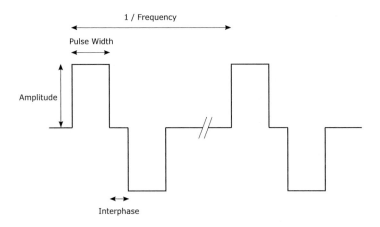

Fig. 2.7. Biphasic stimulation pulse.

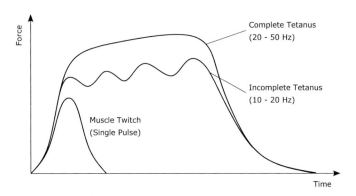

Fig. 2.8. Muscle twitch, incomplete tetanus and complete tetanus.

To avoid an early onset of muscle fatigue or discomfort the frequency is in most cases chosen as low as possible, while still producing a smooth movement.

Amplitude and Pulse Width

Stimulation pulses used for electrical stimulation have a certain amplitude and pulse width (Figure 2.7). The amplitude represents the amount of current in mA delivered to the patient. The pulse width is the duration of the stimulation pulse in µs. Sometimes the pulse width is used to indicate the complete duration of a biphasic stimulation pulse. Here, the pulse width always refers to the duration of the stimulation pulse.

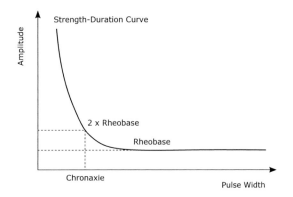

Fig. 2.9. Strength-duration curve.

The electric charge of a stimulation pulse is determined by the product of the amplitude and the pulse width. The combinations of amplitude and pulse width sufficient to elicit an action potential can be illustrated with a strength-duration curve (Figure 2.9). The Rheobase indicates the least amount of current sufficient to elicit an action potential or a muscle response. The Chronaxie is the pulse width where an amplitude of two times the Rheobase leads to a neural response.

Typically, pulse widths are already programmed in the stimulation device and the operator adjusts the amplitude until the desired stimulation effect is achieved. In most cases pulse widths of 250 µs or higher are used. Stimulation with short pulse widths below 100 µs is also possible but requires higher amplitudes.

2.2.3 Electrode Size and Placement

An accurate position of electrodes is crucial for a successful employment of electrical stimulation. The active electrode has to be placed precisely above the motor axons innervating the target muscle. The optimal location to place an active electrode is called motor point. At this point the desired movement can be produced with the least amount of current. It is also possible to place the active electrode over a nerve bundle and stimulate all contained motor axons, leading to contractions of all innervated muscles.

In common practice the indifferent electrode is placed on areas where no stimulation effect is expected (e.g. the wrist for stimulation of forearm muscles). Active electrodes are typically smaller than indifferent electrodes. Small electrodes achieve higher current densities which lead to an easier activation of motor axons. Additionally, a more focal stimulation is possible, allowing to target specific muscles more easily. However, very small electrodes may cause discomfort or pain due to the high current densities. Larger electrodes require higher currents to cause muscle contractions and the stimulation is less focal, potentially activating adjacent muscle groups. Larger electrodes are chosen as indifferent electrodes to reduce the likelihood of unwanted neural activations.

2.2.4 Multi-Channel Electrical Stimulation

To achieve more complex movements like grasping or even walking multiple muscles or muscle groups have to be activated in an orchestrated manner. Therefore, multiple stimulation sites have to be utilized. This can be achieved with multi-channel stimulation devices. One stimulation channel is thereby a pair of active and indifferent electrode. Stimulation parameters like amplitude and pulse width can be adjusted for each channel individually, some devices even allow to utilize multiple stimulation frequencies.

Systems enabling the stimulation of muscle groups to achieve a functional coordinated movement are often called neuroprosthesis, even though technically speaking these systems are generally a orthesis, e.g. a sleeve containing electrodes and potentially sensors.

2.2.5 Limitations

As already mentioned is precise electrode placement a key requirement for successful electrical stimulation. Misplacing electrodes prevents the desired motion to occur and can even cause unwanted movements by activating wrong muscle groups. Even for trained professionals the correct placement of electrodes is not always an easy and obvious task. Therapists tend to place active electrodes always on the muscle belly, even though the motor point may be located somewhere else. Mobile pen-electrodes can be utilized by therapists for a precise determination of effective stimulation points [30] but may overexert patients. Especially when more complex movements involving several stimulation channels shall be performed, the procedure of appropriate electrode placement quickly becomes a tedious task.

Another major limitation of electrical stimulation is the rapid onset of neuromuscular fatigue. During voluntary muscle contractions smaller motor units are activated first. They have a higher fatigue resistance compared to larger motor units that are necessary for higher force generation. Electrical stimulation activates motor units according to their distance from the active electrode and the motor axon diameter. Predominantly large motor axons located close to the active electrode are excited. Motor units are activated simultaneously during electrical stimulation by each pulse and with a frequency that is higher compared to motor unit activation during voluntary contractions. Activation of motor units during normal movements happens in unsynchronized and effective patterns, giving single motor units more time to rest. To offset fatigue more motor units can be activated or the activation rate increased.

Including electrical stimulation in real-life applications to improve the quality of life for stroke survivors suffering from an impaired hand function would require intuitive control methods that are not existent in commercially available systems. Systems that are presented in literature are often complicated and difficult to use for laymen without a technical background.

3 Simulating Neuromuscular Electrical Stimulation

The idea to simulate and calculate the response of tissue to electrical stimulation is not new and has attracted considerable interest over the last decades. Many results are based on the pioneer work of Hodgkin and Huxley [31], who studied the emergence and propagation of action potentials and were rewarded with a Nobel Prize for their work in 1963.

Simulating electrical stimulation is a valuable addition to experimental data and animal models. It can be used to obtain a deeper understanding of the underlying physiological processes. Such a deep understanding is necessary when improvement and innovation is sought. Simulations can be used to assist in two major tasks related to electrical stimulation. First, improving the efficiency of stimulation pulses is a typical field of application. Second, studying the impact of geometrical factors like electrode placement can be done easily.

In this chapter the basic principles for modeling and simulation of electrical stimulation which were used in this thesis will be explained. Further interested readers are invited to refer to the main references, pointed out at the beginning of the relevant sections.

3.1 Two-Step Approach

In this thesis a so called two-step-approach was used to model and simulate neuronal responses caused by electrical stimulation. Such a two-step approach to simulate transcutaneous electrical stimulation was described in detail in [32]. During the first step the electrical potential caused by stimulation pulses in a 3D finite element (FE) model is simulated. The FE model forms a volume conductor supposed to represent a body part or limb, e.g. a human forearm. The actual response of neural tissue, e.g. motor axons, is then calculated in another program using mathematical axon models based on equivalent circuits.

3.2 Finite Element Modeling

The finite element method (FEM) is a numerical method to solve partial differential equations that describe a complex engineering phenomenon. Therefore, a large problem is divided into smaller finite elements. The solution of all these finite elements form the solution of the whole system [33].

In this section the generation of finite element (FE) models, suited for simulation of electrical stimulation, will be explained.

3.2.1 Electric Potential Calculation

COMSOL Multiphysics 4.3 (COMSOL) was used to calculate the electric potential caused by external stimuli in a volume conductor. More precisely the Alternating current/direct current (AC/DC) module was utilized. In COMSOL Maxwell's equations in differential form are solved with respect to certain boundary conditions that are provided by the user. One example of such boundary conditions is the definition of active and indifferent electrodes placed on the simulated volume. The indifferent electrode can be defined as a current source and the active electrode as ground, or vice versa. The necessary information for the two-step approach is the electric potential in close vicinity to the observed motor axon. In COMSOL the transient scalar potential V in a volume conductor is calculated by equation 3.1:

$$-\nabla(\sigma\nabla V + \epsilon_0\epsilon_r\nabla\frac{\partial V}{\partial t}) = 0 \tag{3.1}$$

with σ being the electric conductivity, ϵ_r the relative permittivity and ϵ_0 the electric field constant.

A detailed explanation of the mathematics behind the simulations performed in COMSOL can be found in [34].

3.2.2 Model Geometry

A great advantage of FE models is the possibility to create complex geometries and to change and adjust them easily. Equivalent circuits that describe a volume conductor to represent a limb [35] cannot be adjusted easily and are not suitable to study problems related to electrode geometries and axon orientation. Instead, they offer fast computation times for first approximations.

This study is focused on the investigation of functional electrical stimulation of the hand. Therefore, the model geometry should resemble the human forearm. The main nerves and muscles involved in finger movement are located in the forearm, not directly in the hand. Hence, it is sufficient to model the forearm without the hand (Figure 3.1).

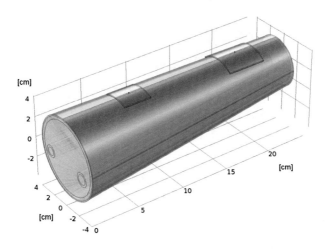

Fig. 3.1. Finite element model of the forearm.

To design a realistic model of a human limb different tissues have to be included, such as: skin, fat, muscle and bones. Moreover, electrodes or a electrode skin interface should be added to simulate the effects of externally applied stimuli (Figure 3.2). All these entities are represented by domains that have specific electrical characteristics. Axons or nerves are much smaller compared to the entire geometry of a human limb and are therefore not present in the FE model. Axons have a thin diameter of a few μm and an even thinner membrane. Thus, modeling these structures would require very small finite elements which would lead to a number of necessary finite elements too high for COMSOL to handle.

According to equation 3.1 σ and ϵ_r have to be known to determine the electric potential V. Therefore, these parameters have to be defined for each domain, representing a different tissue or material. With this information and a given stimulus the potential in the volume conductor can be computed (Figure 3.3).

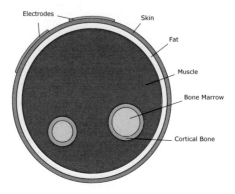

Fig. 3.2. Cross section of the arm with tissues that are included in the simulations.

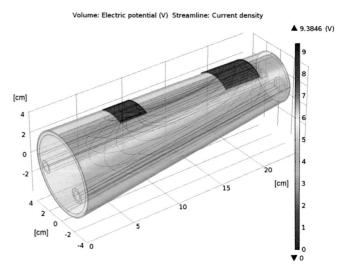

Fig. 3.3. Finite element model of the arm after simulating a response to an external stimulus.

3.2.3 Mesh Dimensions

Mesh settings determine the shape size and number of finite elements. They can be adjusted for each domain separately allowing precise calculations in regions of interest, e.g. in close vicinity to motor axons. Fine meshes result in a higher number of elements which causes long computation times. Hence, it is important to find a balance between accuracy and speed. Increasing the number of finite elements just in regions of interest and keeping the mesh in other areas course can help to achieve such a balance. Another possibility is using a course mesh but to smooth the exported electric potential afterwards in an external program. Figure 3.4 shows the FE model with two different meshes.

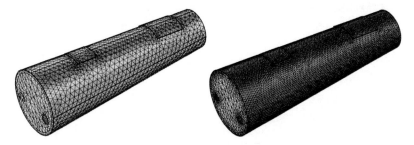

Fig. 3.4. Two differently meshed finite element models. The left model has 31519 elements and had a simulation time of 1 minute and 30 seconds. The right model consists of 186200 elements and the simulation took 13 minutes and 26 seconds.

3.2.4 Model Parameters

Conductivity and permittivity values for different kinds of tissue are provided in COMSOL. Simulations can be performed in the time or frequency domain. For simulations in the frequency domain conductivity and permittivity values have to be provided for each considered frequency. Typically simulations are performed in the time domain with constant electric characteristics. Often simulations of neural stimulation are performed with purely resistive models [36] which offer a sufficient accuracy for stimulation pulses in the range from 25 μs to 1 ms [37].

Kuhn et al. performed a literature review and stimulation experiments with surface and needle electrodes to determine conductivity and permittivity values for a multi-layer volume conductor model of the arm (Table 3.1) [38]. The values obtained by Kuhn

Tab. 3.1. Resistivities and relative permittivities of different tissue layers according to
[38]. Min and Max represent extreme values from [39, 40, 41, 42].

		Min	Standard	Max
Electrode-skin interface	ρ [Ωm]		300	
	ϵ_r	1	1	$2 \cdot 10^6$
Skin	ρ [Ωm]	500	700	$6 \cdot 10^3$
	ϵ_r	$1 \cdot 10^3$	$6 \cdot 10^3$	$30 \cdot 10^3$
Fat	ρ [Ωm]	10	33	600
	ϵ_r	$1 \cdot 10^3$	$25 \cdot 10^3$	$50 \cdot 10^3$
Muscle (axial)	ρ [Ωm]	2	3	5
	ϵ_r	$100 \cdot 10^3$	$120 \cdot 10^3$	$2,5 \cdot 10^6$
Muscle (radial)	ρ [Ωm]	6	9	15
	ϵ_r	$33 \cdot 10^3$	$40 \cdot 10^3$	$830 \cdot 10^3$
Cortical bone	ρ [Ωm]	40	50	60
	ϵ_r		$3 \cdot 10^3$	
Bone marrow	ρ [Ωm]	10	12.5	15
	ϵ_r		$10 \cdot 10^3$	

et al. were used for most simulations performed in this thesis, although, they can be
changed easily. Kuhn showed in his dissertation [21] that the axon excitation threshold
is only influenced a little by the permittivity of the tissue layers. The conductivity of
muscle tissue has a more prominent impact on axon activation, the conductivity of skin
and fat on the other hand only shows a small influence. Due to the smaller conductivity
of skin and fat compared to muscle tissue current flows perpendicular through these
layers, hence, the conductivity only effects the voltage drop and not the current distribution. As long as the simulation of axon excitation is the main goal very accurate
electric parameters of the FE model are of minor importance.

Simplifications

Even though FE models offer many advantages they are of course distinctive simplifications of reality. The simplified geometry and electric parameters as well as the
abundance of inhomogeneities and structures like blood vessels and glands are factors
that distinguish reality from models described in this thesis. Still, many questions re-

lated to the interaction of electrical current and the human body can be investigated to a great extent with the help of 3D representations of limbs and body parts achieved through FE models.

3.3 Axon Models

In 1976 McNeal proposed a model to compute the excitation behavior of myelinated axons to electrical stimuli with a finite duration and electrodes with arbitrary position and geometry [43]. His work was based on the results of Hodgkin and Huxley [31] and Frankenhauser and Huxley [44]. In conjunction with finite element modeling axon models enable the simulation of electrical stimulation.

In this section two variations of this axon model will be presented that were used in this thesis: a passive axon model, neglecting the influence on voltage controlled ion channels and an active model, considering ion channels and describing the course of action potentials. The axon models used in this thesis were implemented in Matlab (MATLAB R2013b, The MathWorks Inc., Natick, Massachusetts, USA).

3.3.1 Passive Axon Model

To allow fast and easy computations several simplifications are made. First, the myelin sheath is considered as a perfect insulator, thereby reducing the number of model elements. Additionally, a constant geometry and constant electric parameters of the motor axons are assumed. Moreover, the electric potential at one node of Ranvier is considered to be constant over the nodal surface.

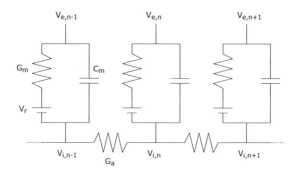

Fig. 3.5. Electrical equivalent circuit of a myelinated axon.

The motor axon equivalent circuit depicted in Figure 3.5 is utilized to compute the membrane potential at a specific node of Ranvier. A capacitance C_m in parallel to a conductance G_m represent the membrane impedance. Applying Kirchhoff's current law to the equivalent circuit from Figure 3.5 leads to Equation 3.2.

$$0 = C_m \frac{d(V_{m,n})}{dt} + G_a(V_{i,n} - V_{i,n-1}) + G_a(V_{i,n} - V_{i,n+1}) + I_n$$

$$0 = C_m \frac{d(V_{m,n})}{dt} + G_a(-V_{i,n-1} + 2V_{i,n} - V_{i,n+1}) + I_n \qquad (3.2)$$

$V_{m,n}$ denotes the membrane potential as $V_{i,n} - V_{e,n} - V_r$, where $V_{i,n}$ is the potential in the inside of the axon and $V_{e,n}$ the extracellular potential, both at the node of Ranvier n. For passive axons the nodal current I_n is simplified to $G_m V_{m,n}$, which corresponds to the subthreshold potential of the membrane, before ion channels start to open, thus, resulting in Equation 3.3.

$$\frac{dV_{m,n}}{dt} = \frac{1}{C_m}[G_a(V_{m,n-1} - 2V_{m,n} + V_{m,n+1} + V_{e,n-1} - 2V_{e,n} + V_{e,n+1}) - G_m V_{m,n}] \quad (3.3)$$

Solving this set of linear differential equations allows the calculation of the motor axon membrane potential as a function of time at any node of Ranvier n. To model axon excitation a threshold potential has to be defined which needs to be surpassed for an activation of the considered axon to occur. In Figure 3.6 the change in membrane potential caused by a 250 µs stimulation pulse, computed with a passive axon model, is shown at one node of Ranvier, located directly under a transcutaneous active electrode. The extracellular potential along the motor axon V_e, used for the computation, was exported from a FE model (Section 3.2).

Typical axon parameters used for this kind of computations are listed in Table 3.2. These values are also used for the simulations shown in the Figures 3.6, 3.8, 3.9, 3.10 and 3.11.

Activating Function

With his publications from 1986 and 1988 Frank Rattay established the term activating function [46, 47]. His work was based on the model from McNeal [43] and utilized the dependance of the membrane potential on the course of the extracellular potential.

By rewriting Equation 3.3 with G_m, G_a and C_m as

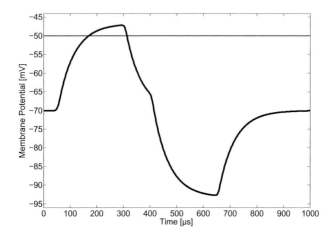

Fig. 3.6. Membrane potential caused by a biphasic stimulation pulse (10 mA, 250 µs, 100 µs interphase), calculated with a passive axon model. Axon parameters are listed in Table 3.2. The axon was located 8 mm beneath the active electrode.

$$G_m = g_m \pi dL \tag{3.4}$$

$$G_a = \frac{\pi d^2}{4\rho_i \Delta x} \tag{3.5}$$

$$C_m = c_m \pi dL \tag{3.6}$$

with g_m and c_m as the membrane conductance and capacitance per unit area, ρ_i the specific axoplasm resistance, L the nodal length and Δx the nodal distance (Figure 3.7) one obtains Equation 3.7.

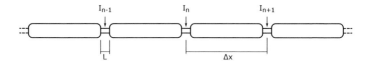

Fig. 3.7. Motor axon with nodal currents.

Tab. 3.2. Typical axon parameters used for the computation of membrane potentials. For the simulations shown in this chapter the internodal distance and axon diameter were chosen as: $\Delta x = 1.5\,$mm and $d = 10\,\mu$m.

Parameter	Value	Reference
internodal distance Δx	1-2 mm	-
node length L	2.5 μm	[43]
axon diameter d	7-17 μm	[45]
specific axoplasm resistance ρ_i	0.7 Ωm	[32]
membrane conductance/unit area g_m	30.4 mS/cm^2	[43]
membrane capacitance/unit area c_m	2 μF/cm^2	[43]
resting potential V_r	-70 mV	[43]
threshold potential V_s	-50 or -55 mV	-

$$\frac{dV_{m,n}}{dt} = \frac{1}{c_m}\left[\frac{d}{4\rho_i}\left(\frac{V_{m,n-1} - 2V_{m,n} + V_{m,n+1}}{\Delta x L} + \frac{V_{e,n-1} - 2V_{e,n} + V_{e,n+1}}{\Delta x L}\right) - g_m V_{m,n}\right] \quad (3.7)$$

Introducing the space constant $\lambda = \sqrt{d/4\rho_i g_m}$ and the time constant $\tau = C_m/G_m = c_m/g_m$ Equation 3.7 simplifies to Equation 3.8.

$$\tau\frac{dV_{m,n}}{dt} - \lambda^2\frac{V_{m,n-1} - 2V_{m,n} + V_{m,n+1}}{\Delta x L} + V_{m,n} = \lambda^2\frac{V_{e,n-1} - 2V_{e,n} + V_{e,n+1}}{\Delta x L} \quad (3.8)$$

At this point it can already be seen that the membrane potential change is proportional to the variation of the extracellular potential along the axon. For a non-myelinated axon one can substitute the nodal distance L with Δx resulting in Equation 3.9.

$$\tau\frac{dV_{m,n}}{dt} - \lambda^2\frac{V_{m,n-1} - 2V_{m,n} + V_{m,n+1}}{\Delta x^2} + V_{m,n} = \lambda^2\frac{V_{e,n-1} - 2V_{e,n} + V_{e,n+1}}{\Delta x^2} \quad (3.9)$$

In the non-myelinated case Δx approaches 0, as a consequence the terms containing Δx^2 in the denominator correspond to the second symmetric derivative, finally leading to Equation 3.10.

$$\tau \frac{\partial V_{m,n}}{\partial t} - \lambda^2 \frac{\partial^2 V_{m,n}}{\partial x^2} + V_{m,n} = \lambda^2 \frac{\partial^2 V_e}{\partial x^2} \qquad (3.10)$$

The right side of this equation is called activating function (Equation 3.11) and is the term driving the axon excitation.

$$f(x,t) = \lambda^2 \frac{\partial^2 V_e}{\partial x^2} \qquad (3.11)$$

Figure 3.8 depicts the activating function (with $\lambda = 1$) along a motor axon, computed at the same time as the membrane potential in Figure 3.6. Positive values of the activating function correspond to parts of the axon where an depolarization occurs, negative values correspond to a hyperpolarization. An active electrode was placed at x = 5 cm and a bigger indifferent electrode at x = 17 cm (Figure 3.3).

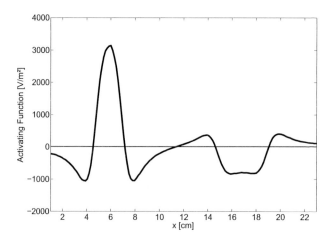

Fig. 3.8. Activating function ($\lambda = 1$) at the end of a 10 mA 250 μs stimulation pulse. The positive peak indicates the region where a depolarization of the membrane occurs (active electrode at x = 5 cm) , negative values correspond to a hyperpolarization indifferent electrode at x = 17 cm. The axon was located 8 mm beneath the active electrode.

Even though the activating function represents the driving term for the activation of non-myelinated axons it can be used for first approximations in the myelinated case. Especially the location of axon activation along the axon and the impact of electrode position and size can estimated with the activating function.

3.3.2 Active Axon Models

To describe the time and voltage dependent course of an action potential the ionic currents that flow through the axon membrane have to be determined. Differential equations computing the ionic currents were first introduced by Hodgkin and Huxley [31] and later by Frankenhaeuser and Huxley [44] alterations [48] or extensions [49, 50] of these equations exist and are still referred to as Hodgkin Huxley like equations. In contrast to passive axon models active axon models contain information about ionic currents and are able to simulate the emergence and propagation of action potentials. Here, the active axon model based on Frankenhaeuser and Huxley (FH) [44] will be presented shortly, as described by McNeal [43]. For active axon models the nodal current is described as the sum of the ionic (sodium and potassium) currents i_{Na}, i_K a nonspecific current i_P and a leakage current i_L (Equation 3.12). The current i_P is a delayed current that is not tied to a specific ion.

$$I = \pi dL(i_{Na} + i_K + i_P + i_L) \tag{3.12}$$

The individual currents can be described with the following set of equations:

$$i_{Na} = \bar{P}_{Na}hm^2\frac{EF^2}{RT}\frac{(Na)_o - (Na)_i e^{EF/RT}}{1 - e^{EF/RT}} \tag{3.13}$$

$$i_K = \bar{P}_K n^2\frac{EF^2}{RT}\frac{(K)_o - (K)_i e^{EF/RT}}{1 - e^{EF/RT}} \tag{3.14}$$

$$i_P = \bar{P}_P p^2\frac{EF^2}{RT}\frac{(Na)_o - (Na)_i e^{EF/RT}}{1 - e^{EF/RT}} \tag{3.15}$$

$$i_L = g_L(V_m - V_L) \tag{3.16}$$

where $E = V_m + V_r$, $\bar{P}_x$ are permeability constants, $(ion)_{o,i}$ the external or internal ion concentrations, R the gas constant, T the temperature and F the Faraday's constant. The variables m, h, n and p are defined as follows:

$$\frac{dm}{dt} = \alpha_m(1-m) - \beta_m m \qquad (3.17)$$

$$\frac{dh}{dt} = \alpha_h(1-h) - \beta_h h \qquad (3.18)$$

$$\frac{dn}{dt} = \alpha_n(1-n) - \beta_n n \qquad (3.19)$$

$$\frac{dp}{dt} = \alpha_p(1-p) - \beta_p p \qquad (3.20)$$

The respective α and β variables can be determined with Equation 3.21. The necessary constants are provided in [44] and [43].

$$(\alpha, \beta)_{m,h,n,p} = a(V_m - b)\left[1 - exp\left(\frac{V_m - c}{d}\right)\right]^{-1} \qquad (3.21)$$

In Figure 3.9 a subthreshold membrane potential computed with an active axon model (FH) is illustrated. Figure 3.10 shows an action potential elicited by an above-threshold stimulation.

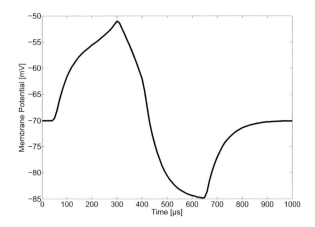

Fig. 3.9. Membrane potential caused by a biphasic subthreshold stimulation pulse (8 mA, 250 µs, 100 µs interphase), calculated with an active axon model according to [44] and [43]. Axon parameters are listed in Table 3.2. The axon was located 8 mm beneath the active electrode.

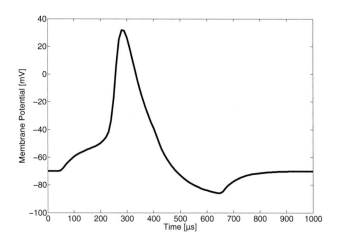

Fig. 3.10. Membrane potential caused by an above-threshold stimulation pulse (10 mA, 250 µs, 100 µs interphase), calculated with an active axon model according to [44] and [43]. Axon parameters are listed in Table 3.2. The axon was located 8 mm beneath the active electrode.

Active axon models can also be used to model the propagation of action potentials along the motor axon, e.g. to investigate the conduction velocity of motor axons or the influence of certain membrane properties on the action potential propagation, as can be seen in Figure 3.11.

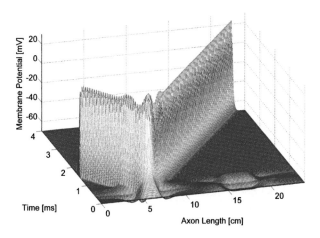

Fig. 3.11. Action potential propagation along an axon. Active axon models enable simulation of action potential propagation along single axons.

3.4 Motor Axon Volume

When FES is performed force is generated by the elicited muscle contractions. The generated force is proportional to the number of activated motor axons. This section will introduce a technique to simulate the activation of multiple motor axons to better understand force generation caused by FES. To perform efficient FES the active electrode should be placed as close as possible to the motor-point. Beneath the motor-point most motor axons are approaching neuromuscular junctions which are spread over the cross section of the muscle. In simple muscles with parallel aligned fibers the neuromuscular junctions are often distributed in a narrow band close to the muscle belly [51]. The motor axon volume (MAV) is supposed to represent the volume which contains the motor axons that approach the neuromuscular junctions. One dominant motor axon orientation is assumed between the area where the nerve enters the muscle and the locations of the neuromuscular junctions. The orientation of the MAV in relation to the forearm model is representing this orientation. The idea behind the motor axon volume is inspired by a publication from Gomez-Tames et al. [45] and is used in section 4.2 to investigate the influence of electrode geometry on force generation during FES. In COMSOL the electric potential in an elliptical cylinder caused by a stimulation pulse is simulated and exported (Figure 3.12).

Homogeneously distributed parallel lines containing the extracellular potential V_e are generated in Matlab with the simulated data from COMSOL. All these lines are representing motor axons with a randomly distributed diameter. For each axon the membrane potential can be calculated with a passive or active axon model as described in previous sections. By calculating the membrane potential for each motor axon it can be determined whether an activation has occurred or not. In case of a passive axon model a predefined threshold voltage has to be surpassed, whereas active axon models require a triggered action potential. Figure 3.13 illustrates the activation of motor axons under the active electrode. In this case a passive axon model was used. It can be seen that motor axons are activated more easily when they have a large diameter and are located close to the active electrode.

The here presented approach allows to visualize the amount of motor axons activated during a stimulation pulse (Figure 3.14 (a)). The diameter distribution of the motor axons has been taken from [45] (Figure 3.14 (b)).

Instead of homogeneously distributed parallel lines it is also possible to generate curves that are located in the MAV. These curves can be distributed randomly in the MAV.

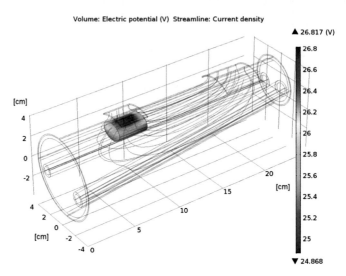

Fig. 3.12. 3D finite element model of the human forearm. The red lines represent the current flow between the active and indifferent electrode, the multicolored volume illustrates the electric potential in the motor axon volume caused by a monophasic stimulation pulse (20 mA, 250 μs).

Curved motor axons may provide a more accurate representation of the actual anatomy. The extracellular potential along the motor axons is then determined via a 3D interpolation. However, a higher resolution of the exported data is required for the interpolation to obtain good results. Furthermore, a continuous shape of the motor axons is important to prevent spikes in the activating function, resulting in to early activations. Figure 3.15 shows the activation of curved motor axons under the active electrode, a passive axon model was used again to determine axon activation.

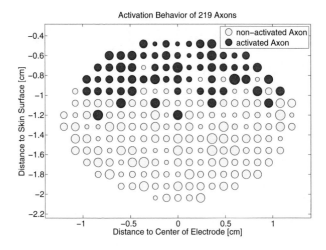

Fig. 3.13. Cross section of the motor axon volume. Red circles represent activated motor axons, yellow ones represent non-activated motor axons. The size of the circles corresponds to the actual diameter of the motor axon.

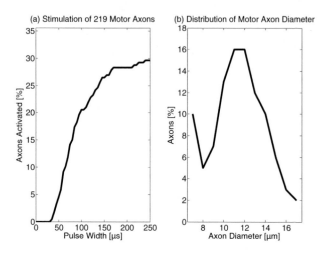

Fig. 3.14. Activation of motor axons during a stimulation pulse (a). With increasing time more and more axons are activated. Axon activation was assumed when a threshold voltage (here -55 mV) was surpassed in a passive axon model. Distribution of motor axon diameters in the motor axon volume (b) [45].

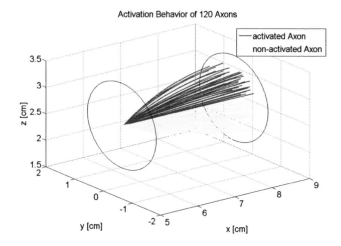

Fig. 3.15. Motor axon volume with curved axons located beneath the active electrode. The axons share one point of origin.

3.5 Pulse Response Calculation

Computation time can be a limiting factor when working with 3D FE models. Especially when different pulseforms are supposed to be investigated many simulations become necessary. For that reason, a method was developed to avoid multiple simulations in COMSOL, allowing the adjustment of the pulsform directly in Matlab. The 3D FE model represents a linear time-invariant (LTI) system, hence, the response to a short pulse of the system can be used to calculate its response to any excitation which can be described as a linear combination of such short pulses. For this purpose the response $V(t)$ to a short rectangular pulse (1 mA, 1 μs) is superimposed to obtain the system response $V_{stim}(t)$ to an arbitrary stimulus $x_{stim}(t)$. The unit less vector $x_{stim}(t)$ describes the arbitrary stimulus as a linear combination of the short rectangular pulse which led to the response $V(t)$, e.g. at a node of Ranvier. If the potential at a node of Ranvier is investigated the vector V_{stim} corresponds to the extracellular potential $V_{e,n}$ caused at a specific node of Ranvier n (see section 3.3).

$$\vec{V}_{stim} = K \ \vec{x}_{stim} \tag{3.22}$$

with $K =$

$$\begin{pmatrix} V(t_0) & 0 & \dots & 0 \\ V(t_1) & V(t_0) & \dots & 0 \\ \vdots & \vdots & \ddots & \vdots \\ V(t_{end}) & V(t_{end-1}) & \dots & V(t_0) \end{pmatrix}$$

The columns of matrix K (unit = V) contain the shifted pulse response of the system which is illustrated in Figure 3.16. A matrix vector multiplication can then be used to obtain the response to another stimulus (Figure 3.17).

In Figure 3.18 a comparison of a classical stimulation response exported from COMSOL and one computed with a pulse response in Matlab is illustrated. Only a small deviation can be observed due to small distortions of the short rectangular pulse in COMSOL. However, such a small deviation does not affect the qualitative results that

K

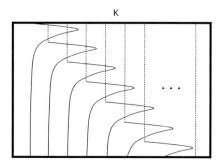

Fig. 3.16. Visualization of matrix K. The columns of matrix K contain the shifted pulse response of the system.

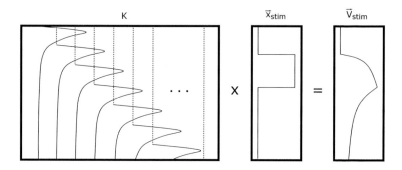

Fig. 3.17. Multiplication of matrix K and vector $\vec{x}_{stim}$, containing an arbitrary stimulus, yields the system response $\vec{V}_{stim}$. $\vec{V}_{stim}$ shows the electric potential at a specific point in the FE model elicited by an external stimulus $\vec{x}_{stim}$.

shall be obtained with this sort of approach.

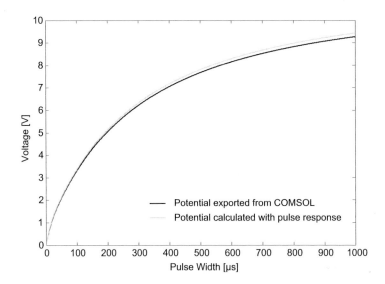

Fig. 3.18. Comparison of electric potential caused by a 1 ms stimulation pulse exported from COMSOL and computed with a pulse response in Matlab.

This approach can be used to calculate the extracellular potential along a motor axon at every node of Ranvier. The main advantage of this method is that the number of computational demanding simulations can be reduced significantly. New simulations are only necessary when the electric parameters or the geometry of the FE model are altered. Furthermore, utilizing the LTI behavior of the system allows the execution of optimization algorithms (Section 4.1.1).

4 Considerations for Efficient Electrical Stimulation

In this chapter several considerations regarding efficient electrical stimulation will be discussed. Many of these are based on the information provided in Chapter 3 as well as practical trials performed at the Institute of Nano- and Medical Electronics at the Hamburg University of Technology. At the beginning the efficiency of single stimulation pulses will be examined followed by an investigation of the impact of electrode geometry on force generation during FES. After that the presentation of possibilities to utilize and fabricate array electrodes will finalize the chapter. Later on in Chapter 7 findings from experimental studies, which were heavily influenced by the considerations shown in the following chapter, will be presented.

4.1 Stimulation Pulse Efficiency

Many studies have investigated whether stimulation pulses different from rectangular ones can provide a more efficient stimulation or not [52, 53, 54, 55, 56]. Most of them focused on energy minimization. Current controlled stimulation pulses are typically provided through a constant high voltage source in the stimulation device. The maximum stimulation current that can be achieved depends on the resistance between the stimulation electrodes. With a constant voltage source in the stimulation device the energy consumption of a single stimulation pulse depends solely on the product of the amplitude and pulse width which is equivalent to the electric charge of the stimulation pulse. Moreover, less electric charge per pulse can also lead to less stress for the patient and a smaller likelihood of tissue damage due to charge accumulation beneath the electrodes.

In this section the charge optimization of stimulation pulse will be described. Additionally, the influence of a stimulation interphase on the activation amplitude and the effect of pulse width on selectivity will be addressed shortly.

4.1.1 Charge Optimization

In Section 3.5 a method to determine the response of a FE model to an arbitrary electrical stimulus by exploiting the linear time invariant character of the system was presented. Here, this approach is extended to determine the membrane potential of an motor axon, again using a pulse response. Experiences from preliminary experiments have led to the assumption that there might be a correlation between charge and stimulation pulse efficiency as well the stimulation comfort. The here presented theoretical simulation study was supposed to support these assumptions and was presented at the Biodevices 2016 [57].

At first the extracellular potential caused by a short rectangular pulse ($1\,\mathrm{mA}$, $1\,\mathrm{\mu s}$) along a line was exported from COMSOL. This potential was used in Matlab to compute the membrane potential at every node of Ranvier of a motor axon with a passive axon model. The membrane potential at the investigated node of Ranvier $V_m(t)$ was superimposed to obtain the system response $V_{m,stim}(t)$ to an arbitrary stimulus $x_{stim}(t)$.

$$\vec{V}_{m,stim} = G\,\vec{x}_{stim} \tag{4.1}$$

with $G =$

$$\begin{pmatrix} V_m(t_0) & 0 & \cdots & 0 \\ V_m(t_1) & V_m(t_0) & \cdots & 0 \\ \vdots & \vdots & \ddots & \vdots \\ V_m(t_{end}) & V_m(t_{end-1}) & \cdots & V_m(t_0) \end{pmatrix}$$

The columns of matrix G contain the shifted membrane potential caused by the short rectangular pulse at one node of Ranvier. In Matlab a minimization problem was solved to minimize the electric charge of the stimulation pulse $x_{stim}(t)$ which is required to cause the membrane potential to surpass the activation threshold:

$$\int_0^{t_{end}} x_{stim}(t)\,\mathrm{d}t \rightarrow min \tag{4.2}$$

with t_{end} being the last observed point of time and thus, also the maximum allowed pulse width.

In Matlab the minimization problem was treated as a linear programming problem. The formulation of this linear programming problem is unfortunately not intuitive. At the beginning boundary conditions had to be provided. The stimulation pulse was not allowed to exceed a duration of $t_{end} = 500\,\mu s$. Additionally, a maximum amplitude (a_{max}) of the stimulation pulse was set. Most importantly, the activation threshold had to be surpassed at $t = t_{end}$ but not before. Now, the minimization problem was actually turned into a maximization problem, by defining an initial solution $\vec{x}_{start}$ that reached the threshold potential at t_{end}. A rectangular pulse with a duration of $500\,\mu s$ and an amplitude of a_{start} was used as the starting solution, since it is well known that long duration rectangular pulses require a lot of charge for axon activation [58]. The linear programming solver searched a solution for the objective $\vec{x} = \vec{x}_{start} - \vec{x}_{stim}$ to be as big as possible, thus, minimizing $\vec{x}_{stim}$. The final formulation used for the computation in Matlab can be seen here:

$$\min_{\vec{x}} \vec{f}^T \vec{x} \text{ such that } \begin{cases} A\,\vec{x} \leq \vec{b}, \\ lb(t) \leq x(t) \leq ub(t). \end{cases} \tag{4.3}$$

with $\vec{x} = \vec{x}_{start} - \vec{x}_{stim}$, $lb(t) = x_{start}(t) - a_{max}$, $ub(t) = x_{start}(t)$, $\vec{f} = [-1, -1, ..., -1]^T$, $\vec{b} = [0, 0, ..., 0]^T$ and $A =$

$$\begin{pmatrix} -V_m(t_0) & 0 & \cdots & 0 \\ -V_m(t_1) & -V_m(t_0) & \cdots & 0 \\ \vdots & \vdots & \ddots & \vdots \\ +V_m(t_{end}) & +V_m(t_{end-1}) & \cdots & +V_m(t_0) \end{pmatrix}$$

Figure 4.1 illustrates the results of the minimization problem for maximum amplitudes of 20, 40 and 60 mA. It can be seen that the optimal solutions resemble rectangular pulses that use the maximum available stimulation amplitude. Higher maximum amplitudes lead to lower electric charge. Short stimulation pulses were reported to be most charge efficient [55, 58], which is in line with the finding presented here. It is interesting to note that no other pulse shape outperformed a rectangular one in terms of charge efficiency. An experimental comparison of short (60 µs) and long (300 µs) stimulation pulses based on the results of this chapter is presented in Section 7.2.

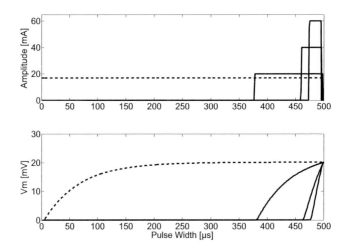

Fig. 4.1. Optimized stimulation pulses and the respective membrane potentials (V_m). The dashed line represents the initial solution and membrane potential.

4.1.2 Stimulation Interphase

Biphasic stimulation pulses do often have an interphase to avoid a negative effect of the reverse pulse on the stimulation outcome. The effect of the interphase duration was assessed with an active axon model for three different pulse widths (60, 180 and 300 µs). Figure 4.2 exhibits the normalized activation amplitude depending on the interphase duration. A greater effect of the interphase was observed for short pulse widths. An interphase of 200 µs was sufficient to avoid any effect for all three pulse widths. 100 µs reduced the increase in necessary amplitude to below 5 %.

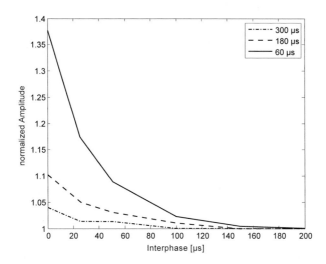

Fig. 4.2. Normalized activation amplitude over interphase duration. The amplitudes for each pulse width were normalized with its value at 200 µs. The necessary amplitude increases when short or no interphases between the cathodic and anodic pulses are used. The effect is stronger for short pulse width. With an 100 µs interphase the amplitude increase is less than 5 %.

4.1.3 Stimulation Pulse Selectivity

Grill et al. reported how short pulse width stimulation allows a more spatially selective stimulation of motor axons at specific depths [59]. These results were verified and extended to judge whether short pulse width also allow a more selective stimulation of motor axons with different diameters.

Figure 4.3 shows strength-duration curves for motor axons at different depths in the tissue. The absolute difference between curves is increasing for shorter pulse widths, whereas the relative difference remains more or less the same.

Figure 4.4 shows strength-duration curves for motor axons with different diameters. Similar to Figure 4.3 the absolute difference between curves is increasing for shorter pulse widths, whereas the relative difference remains more or less the same.

Larger absolute differences and higher necessary stimulation amplitudes result in an easier grading of stimulation outcome and a higher selectivity. The amplitude can be

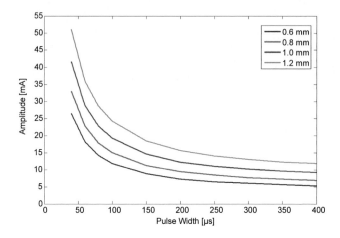

Fig. 4.3. Strength-duration curves for different axon depths. Axons with a higher
distance to the active electrode require higher currents to be activated. The
absolute difference of the required current between different axon depths
increases for short pulse widths.

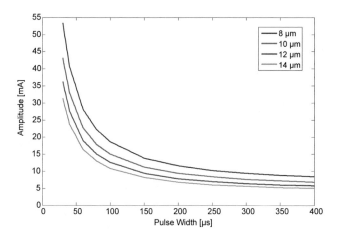

Fig. 4.4. Strength-duration curves for different axon diameters. Axons with a smaller
diameter require higher currents to be activated. The absolute difference of
the required current between different axon diameters increases for short
pulse widths.

adjusted stepwise in order to activate more fibers at different depths or with different diameters and thus allow a precise control of muscle contraction strength.

4.2 Impact of Electrode Geometry

Electrode arrays contain many single electrodes which can be designed in various different shapes. In this section the question how single electrodes in an electrode array should look like will be investigated. The placement and geometry of electrodes has a direct influence on the electric field generated by electrical stimulation. Also, the alignment of motor axons to this electric field determines their likelihood to be activated by stimulation pulses. The activating function is a simple tool to make first estimations of the impact of electrode geometry on axon activation. For a given current and electrode area the peak of the activating function decreases considerably if the electrode is aligned parallel to the motor axon, corresponding to a lower depolarization of the membrane potential (Figure 4.5).

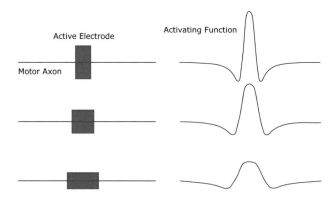

Fig. 4.5. Schematic illustration of the activating function beneath active electrodes with different geometries. Electrode area and current density are constant for all three scenarios.

To better understand how this behavior effects force generation during FES a simulation study and experiments with two healthy subjects were performed. This study was published [60] and the results were presented at the 49th annual conference of the German Society for Biomedical Engineering.

4.2.1 Simulation

For the simulation a simple 3D FE model (COMSOL) of the human forearm was used (Figure 4.6). The electric parameters of the FE model can be seen in Table 4.1. A distal indifferent electrode (4 x 4 cm^2) and an active electrode were placed on the skin layer. Under the center of the active electrode a 16 mm high, 24 mm wide and 30 mm long MAV (Section 3.4) with an elliptic cross section was located. Estimations of the MAV dimensions were made with regard to [61, 62, 63]. Angles of 0°, 30° and 60° between the MAV and the longitudinal direction of the forearm were examined (Figure 4.7 (a)). A truncated pyramid was used instead of a cylinder or truncated cone for the FE model to allow easy rotation of the MAV.

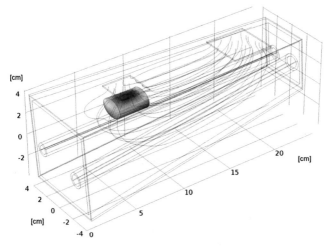

Fig. 4.6. 3D FE model of the human forearm. The red lines represent the current flow between the active and indifferent electrode and the multicolored volume illustrates the electric potential in the motor axon volume. A volume with flat surfaces was chosen to allow easy rotation of the motor axon volume.

A longitudinal placed electrode (2 x 4 cm^2), a transversal placed electrode (4 x 2 cm^2) and a square electrode with an area of 8 cm^2 (Figure 4.7 (b)) were used as active electrodes in this simulation study and in the following experiments. All electrodes geometries have the same center and area. The simulations were performed with monophasic 150 µs, 20 mA stimulation pulses. Biphasic pulses would not alter the results of the simulation but require longer computation time. To evaluate the effectiveness of the different electrode geometries the number of activated motor axons was calculated in Matlab with a passive axon model. Therefore, 219 homogeneously distributed parallel motor axons were generated and it was checked whether the membrane potential ex-

Tab. 4.1. Parameters used for the 3D FE model. The conductivity σ and permittivity ϵ_r are taken from [32]. The geometry of the tissue was estimated.

Material	σ [S/m]	ϵ_r	Thickness [mm]
Electrode-skin interface	1/300	1	1
Skin	1/700	$6 \cdot 10^3$	1.5
Fat	1/33	$25 \cdot 10^3$	2.5
Muscle (axial)	1/3	$120 \cdot 10^3$	240
Muscle (radial)	1/9	$40 \cdot 10^3$	73-43
Cortical bone	1/50	$3 \cdot 10^3$	ca. 2
Bone marrow	2/25	$10 \cdot 10^3$	ca. 8

ceeded a threshold potential (Figure 3.13).

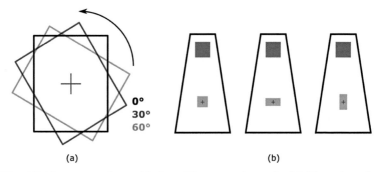

(a)   (b)

Fig. 4.7. Motor axon volume with three different rotation angles (a). Three electrode geometries that were used in the simulation and in the experimental validation (b).

4.2.2 Experimental Validation

To validate the simulation results measurements with two young and healthy subjects were performed. The subjects were seated comfortably at a table with a set up for force measurement in front of them (Figure 4.8). Measurements were performed on the right arm. The arm was placed in a supinated position on the table and fixated. The index, middle and ring finger were attached to a string that was connected via a spring to a force gauge (PCE-FG 20SD, PCE Instruments, Meschede, Germany). Electrode dimension and placement were consistent with the simulations. The indifferent electrode was placed close to the wrist and the active electrodes were placed on the motor point for finger flexion. This motor point was carefully determined by using a pen electrode. All three electrode geometries were centered on the mark of the motor point. Stimulations were performed with biphasic 150 µs stimulation pulses (100 µs interphase) and a frequency of 35 Hz. The amplitude was adjusted to cause a strong and repeatable contraction without causing discomfort (15 mA for subject 1 and 12 mA for subject 2). A sequence of 5 s stimulation followed by a 20 s break was repeated 5 times for each of the three electrode configurations. The peak force for each sequence was noted and the median of all 5 values determined. To avoid fatigue altering the results there was a 5 minute break between each electrode configuration.

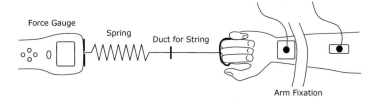

Fig. 4.8. Experimental set up for force measurements. The index, middle and ring finger are attached with a string and a spring to a force gauge.

4.2.3 Results

To evaluate the simulation and experimental results the simulated axon activation and the measured force were normalized. In Figure 4.9 the measurement and simulation results are illustrated. The experimental results between subject 1 and 2 vary a lot. Subject 1 achieved the highest force with a transversal electrode, whereas subject 2 achieved the highest level of force with a longitudinal one. Similar behavior can be seen for the simulation results with differently rotated MAV favoring different electrode configurations. It is interesting to notice that for each subject a different MAV orientation offers a good correlation between experimental and simulated results.

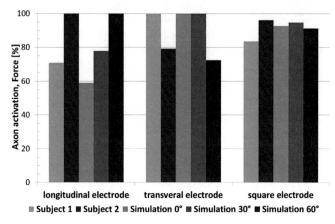

Fig. 4.9. Comparison of experimental with simulation results. The experimental results of subject 1 and 2 are illustrated as normalized force, the simulation results for all motor axon volume orientations are illustrated as the normalized number of activated axons. A longitudinal placed electrode (2 x 4 cm^2), a transversal placed electrode (4 x 2 cm^2) and a square electrode with an area of 8 cm^2 were used for the experiments and simulations. Biphasic stimulation pulses with a pulse width of 150 µs and a 100 µs interphase were used for the experiments (15 mA for subject 1 and 12 mA for subject 2). Simulations were performed with monophasic stimulation pulses with a pulse width of 150 µs and an amplitude of 20 mA.

4.2.4 Conclusion

Even though just two subjects participated in this study the different experimental results observed in conjunction with the simulation study have some interesting implications. Apparently the dominant motor axon orientation can vary strongly from one subject to another. Also the concept of the MAV proved as a useful tool to simulate force generation by electrical stimulation. Rectangular electrodes placed on the skin always have the possibility to be aligned in parallel to the motor axons that are supposed to be stimulated. Thus, over 40 % of stimulation effect can potentially be lost. Square or round electrodes do not have that risk and performed rather well in all scenarios, making them a good choice when the dominant motor axon orientation is unknown. Hence, single electrodes on electrode arrays should be square or round.

4.3 Utilizing Array Electrodes

Array electrodes offer a variety of possibilities to improve FES. The key feature is that the stimulation points can be moved around freely on the array without having to detach and reattach electrodes each time. Here, three techniques exploiting electrode arrays will be introduced.

4.3.1 Automatic Electrode Determination

Array electrodes offer a high number of possible stimulation sites. To use array electrodes efficiently the electrodes on the array producing the desired outcome have to be determined. There are several ways to determine which electrodes should be used. The simplest approach is to activate each electrode successively and evaluate the outcome visually. This could either be done by the patient or a therapist. When a high number of electrodes is used it could be difficult to remember which one produced the best outcome. Sensors quantifying the elicited movement may support or even partly automate this process. Accelerometers [64] and flex sensors [7] have been used successfully to asses stimulation efficiency of stimulation sites on an electrode array. It has to be noted that the hand has multiple degrees of freedom, making a complete assessment of movement induced by electrical stimulation nearly impossible. Flex sensors might record a strong finger extension but cannot recognize a wrist rotation the subject could perceive as unpleasant. Therefore, results provided by sensors should be regarded as suggestions for effective stimulation sites. The final decision should be performed by the patient or therapist. Figure 4.10 illustrates the result of an electrode search program where 14 electrodes were activated successively and the finger extension was measured by flex sensors placed on the fingers.

4.3.2 Virtual Electrodes

Array electrodes offer the possibility to form so called virtual electrodes out of single elements of the array [21]. The current from one stimulation channel is thereby distributed over multiple electrodes instead of a single one (Figure 4.11). In theory this allows to form virtual electrodes specifically shaped or distributed achieving the desired movement [10]. The number of electrodes forming a virtual electrode is determined by the size and number of available electrodes as well as the number of suitable stimulation sites. In a simple scenario two electrodes next to each other on the array can

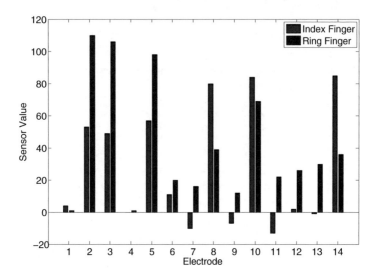

Fig. 4.10. Results of an electrode search program with 14 active electrodes. Flex sensors were used to evaluate the extension of the index and ring finger.

be activated simultaneously to form one bigger electrode (Figure 4.12 A) stimulating the same muscle. It is also possible to use very small electrodes to form more complex shapes and to move the stimulation area precisely (Figure 4.12 B). However, using very small single electrodes could potentially harm the patient if they are activated individually due to high current densities. Moreover, the process of defining and adjusting these stimulation areas can become quite complex objecting the idea to simplify the stimulation process with array electrodes.

Virtual electrodes can also be utilized to achieve certain functional tasks or grasping patterns [10]. In this case stimulation will not compulsively target the same muscle. Stimulation sites may be located centimeters apart over different muscles which are involved in the same movement. However, distributing the current from one stimulation channel over multiple electrodes with different distances to the indifferent electrode will lead to an uneven division of stimulation amplitude. The active electrode closest to the indifferent electrode will have a higher amplitude than more distant ones. Even without this uneven current distribution it can be difficult to adjust the stimulation amplitude appropriately because stimulation of different muscles might require different

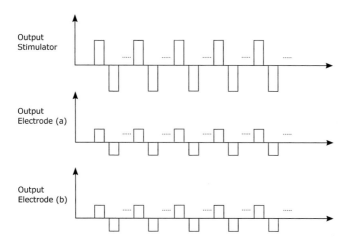

Fig. 4.11. Simultaneous activation of two electrodes connected to one stimulation channel results in a reduced amplitude for each electrode. In an ideal scenario the amplitude would be exactly halved.

amplitudes. With a virtual electrode stimulation intensity cannot be controlled for each element individually. Hence, in most cases multi-channel stimulation should be the method of choice when functional tasks involving several muscles shall be achieved.

4.3.3 Distributed Low Frequency Stimulation

Distributed Low Frequency Stimulation (DLFS) is a technique which utilizes multiple elements on array electrodes in order to reduce muscle fatigue induced by FES. Several variations of this technique have been discussed in literature [65, 66, 67, 68]. As described in Section 2.2.5 rapid occurrence of fatigue during FES is one major limitation in clinical use. DLFS tries to stimulate different motor axons which are innervating the same muscle with a lower frequency than normally used (Figure 4.13). This technique requires the muscle to have more than one effective stimulation site or motor point (Figure 4.14). Then multiple electrodes have to be located over the same muscle and be activated successively. This leads to a less frequent stimulation of the same motor axons, giving them more time to rest. Especially stimulation of big muscles like the Quadriceps is a promising field of application. On the Quadriceps it is likely to find multiple effective stimulation sites and placement of the electrodes is easier. Maneski et al. could show that DLFS can also be used for forearm muscles [69]. This means

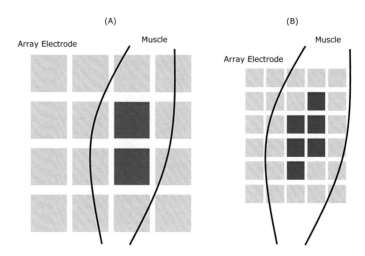

Fig. 4.12. Simple virtual electrode with two elements activated over the target muscle
(A). More complex virtual electrode formed out of six elements over the
target muscle (B).

an application in grasping neuroprosthesis seems possible. However, comparisons were
done to an active electrode much larger than the successively activated ones used for
DLFS [65, 66, 67, 68] or with different pulse rates [69]. To the best of the author's
knowledge it has not been studied how DLFS performs compared to stimulation with
a single small electrode on the array. It might be possible that using just one small
very well placed electrode performs equally well in regard to muscle fatigue.

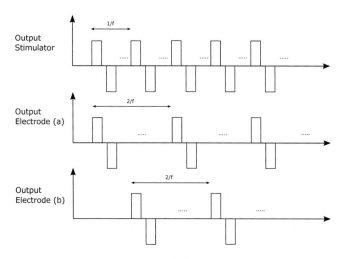

Fig. 4.13. Distributed Low Frequency Stimulation (DLFS) dividing stimulation current on two electrodes. Stimulation frequency at each electrode is thereby reduced by half in this example.

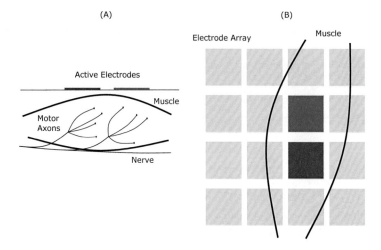

Fig. 4.14. Active electrodes placed over two motor points innervating the same muscle (A). Two electrodes on the electrode array placed over the target muscle are highlighted (B).

4.4 Design and Fabrication of Array Electrodes

Koutsou et al. [70] presented an overview of array electrodes that were used in research activities. The array electrodes were divided in two categories:

1. *Plastic flexible substrate electrodes* based on flexible printed circuit boards.

2. *Textile electrodes* based on knitted conductive yarn or screen printed fabrics.

The first kind of electrodes are based on flexible printed circuit boards (FPCB) and are the most common approach [7, 71, 72, 73]. A pattern of conductive material is applied on a plastic flexible substrate with an insulation layer on top just revealing the parts of the pattern that are supposed to form the single electrodes on the array. An additional hydrogel layer is then used to achieve a good skin contact [74]. The hydrogel layer can consist of many single separated elements without contact between each other or one single sheet, covering the whole array. Single hydrogel elements provide a more focal stimulation by preventing lateral currents through the gel sheet but may also cause higher current densities. Furthermore, the fabrication process of the array electrode becomes considerably more challenging. When a single hydrogel sheet is used the impedance and thickness of the gel as well as the distance between the single electrodes are of mayor importance. A high gel impedance limits lateral current flow [21]. The impact of other highly conductive electrodes attached to the same hydrogel sheet has to be considered to avoid current flowing laterally through the gel and through other electrodes on the array.

Figure 4.15 shows the electric potential caused by stimulation pulse on a simple electrode array with two different hydrogel resistivities. Figure 4.16 shows the corresponding activating functions. A higher resistivity of the hydrogel leads to a stronger more focal excitation.

Another approach to design stimulation electrodes for FES are textile electrodes [75]. Including textiles into neurological rehabilitation activities to sense motion or muscle activity as well as to perform electrical stimulation has gained an increase in interest [76]. Yang et al. [77] presented a method to produce screen printed fabric array electrodes. Such electrodes offer the possibility to be easily integrated into orthesis or clothes. They could also be washed and be even used dry. However, it has been reported that textile electrodes, especially when dry, cause an increased discomfort during stimulation [78].

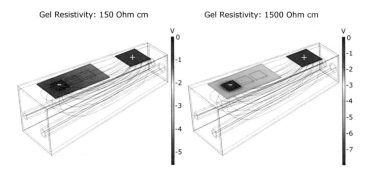

Fig. 4.15. Electric potential caused by a stimulation pulse for two different hydrogel resistivities.

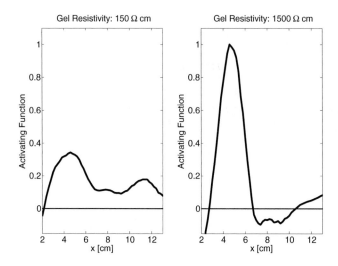

Fig. 4.16. Activating function caused by a stimulation pulse with two different hydrogel resistivities. A higher gel resistivity results in a smaller amount of current flowing laterally through the gel and, thereby, a higher current density under the active electrode.

Even though the potential of textile electrodes is tempting electrodes based on FPCBs were favored in this project, since the development of textile electrodes is still in its initial state and its effectiveness for real-life applications with impaired patients has not yet been proven.

When designing electrode arrays square or round electrode pads were favored over rectangular or elliptic ones due to the results presented in Section 4.2.

4.4.1 Flexible Printed Circuit Board Electrodes

The first electrode arrays designed in this project were flexible printed circuit boards manufactured (LeitOn GmbH, Berlin, Germany) similar to [71]. The surface of the conductive electrode pads is made of electroless nickel immersion gold. Nickel is covered completely by a thin layer of immersion gold which prevents oxidation as well as direct skin contact, making this the electrode suitable for non-permanent transcutaneous applications [71].

4.4.2 Ink-jet printed Array Electrodes

For rapid prototyping a novel technique was developed since the approach described in section 4.4.1 is costly and the delivery time is high. The idea was to establish a fast and cheap prototyping technique to create FPCBs with a commercial ink-jet printer. It has already been shown that ECG electrodes can be manufactured with a similar approach [79].

The whole array electrode consists of a polyester film as the substrate, conductive silver ink, another polyester film with an adhesive side and punched out contacts as insulation and a hydrogel sheet. Instead of the polyester film photographic paper can be used as a substrate as well and provides good contact to the silver ink (Figure 4.19). However, the photographic paper is less durable compared to the polyester film and less resistant to moisture, coming from the hydrogel or sweat. Thus, for long term applications a polyester substrate should be preferred.

Marks for punching out the contacts for the electrode pads should be printed on the insulation layer. Additional marks can help to align the substrate and insulation layer. Since in this prototyping approach the contacts were punched out manually with a 12 mm hollow puncher. The size of the conductive pads on the substrate was chosen larger as the finally used contact area (Figure 4.17) to leave room for some margin of error. Figure 4.18 shows the combined substrate and insulation layer together with a custom made connector.

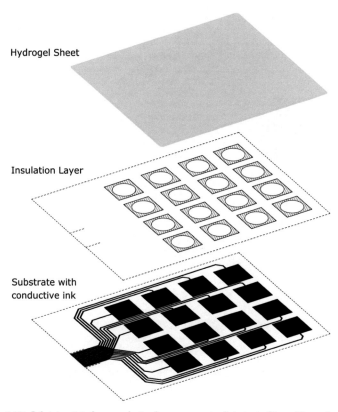

Hydrogel Sheet

Insulation Layer

Substrate with
conductive ink

Fig. 4.17. Ink-jet printed array electrode components. Substrate film with conductive pattern (bottom). Insulation layer with marks to punch out electrode contacts (middle). The marks for the electrode contacts are chosen in a different shape and size compared to the conductive pattern to account for inaccuracy during fabrication. Hydrogel sheet (top).

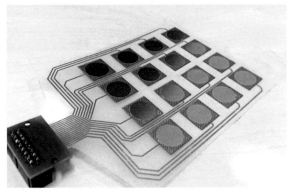

Fig. 4.18. Combined substrate and insulation layer are forming a complete ink-jet printed array electrode. Hydrogel has not yet been attached to the array electrode.

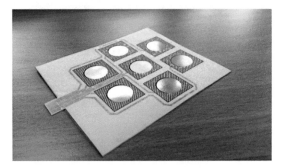

Fig. 4.19. Array electrode fabricated by ink-jet printing with a photographic paper substrate. Hydrogel has not yet been attached to the array electrode.

5 Systems for Electrical Stimulation with Array Electrodes

To use array electrodes a demultiplexer is required to distribute the stimulation current to the desired electrodes on the array (Figure 5.1). The demultiplexer needs to contain switches able to withstand high currents and voltages. During the use of electrical stimulation currents of up to 100 mA and voltages up to 150 V are not a rare occurrence. Therefore, relays were used in literature [80], since they provide a mechanical separation of the target electrode and the current source, making them the most secure solution. This is especially true, if the demultiplexer and the stimulation device are separate systems that are not synchronized in any way.

Two possible approaches to support the use array electrodes will be explained in the following sections. The first is a straight forward concept, featuring a demultiplexer, independent from the stimulation device, thus very flexible. This sort of demultiplexer will from now on be referred to as type I demultiplexer. A stimulation system containing such a type I demultiplexer was developed and will be explained in Section 5.2.

The second approach will explain a more complex concept, featuring a demultiplexer synchronized with the stimulation device (type II demultiplexer). A fully functional prototype will be presented afterwards in Section 5.4.

5.1 Type I Demultiplexers

Neither array electrodes nor stimulation systems supporting them are currently commercially available. To still be able to study electrical stimulation with array electrodes here a simple concept to achieve a first demultiplexer system will be presented.

Working with patients and testing array electrodes in a real life scenario usually re-

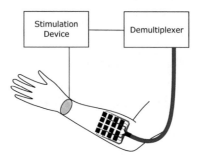

Fig. 5.1. Simple principle of a demultiplexer connected to a stimulation device to utilize array electrodes. The demultiplexer is distributing the current to the array electrode. One indifferent electrode is connected directly to the stimulation device.

quires the use of commercial and certified stimulation devices. Therefore, building a new stimulation device is often out of the question, which would also require a lot of engineering work and know how. That is why the first presented concept will describe flexible stand alone systems that are not synchronized with the stimulation device.

The easiest way to use array electrodes is by utilizing mechanical switches for each electrode. These could either be on/off switches as used by [71] or on/off/on switches. On/off/on switches do even allow to switch between active and indifferent electrodes. Such purely mechanical systems are of course very limited in its functionality and by the number of electrodes that can be controlled reasonably, still they provide a very easy option to distribute stimulation current to multiple electrodes.

A more sophisticated method is to employ relays controlled by a microcontroller or computer. Typically sensors or data gloves are incorporated into electrically controlled demultiplexer a PC is used to control the system over a serial interface [80, 81]. Sensors are a possibility to provide feedback to the system and the user about the effectiveness of the chosen electrodes, preferably to find the most suitable stimulation site on the array.

Type I demultiplexers have no information when single stimulation pulses arrive. Therefore, they have to be capable of prohibiting current flow through the body (Figure 5.2). Many simple stimulation devices have limited control possibilities. Normally predefined stimulation programs are used which do not allow to start and stop stimulation as pleased. Some devices have switch inputs allowing to start stimulation phases at will. Connecting a simple stimulation device without these switch inputs to a type I demultiplexer can provide an additional control layer. The demultiplexer decides when stimulation current is allowed to flow and to which electrode. This works as long as the stimulation device can be set to a continuous stimulation program without pauses. However, this method can be inefficient energy wise as many stimulation pulses might be unused.

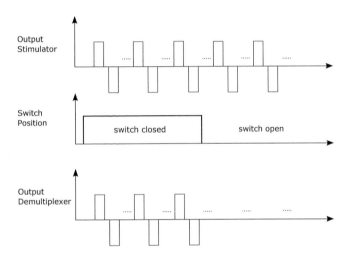

Fig. 5.2. External switches determine when stimulation current is allowed to reach the patient. Closing the switch passes the stimulation current to the associated electrode.

Unfortunately these systems have disadvantages regarding their handling, since it is required to control the stimulation device as well as the demultiplexer. Another major limitation is the difficult use of multiple stimulation channels. Stimulation devices for NMES or FES do typically have between one and eight independent stimulation channels. For many applications one or two channels are sufficient. However, more complex stimulation tasks require a higher channel count. The problem with independent demultiplexers is their lack of knowledge about stimulation pulse timings. When timings are unknown every stimulation channel requires one switch for each electrode used, therefore, multiplying the number of total switches for each desired stimulation channel (Figure 5.3). Stimulation channels may not be allowed to share switches to prevent multiple channels using the same electrode by accident. An eight channel stimulator supposed to use 32 electrodes requires 256 switches, thus making a compact system design nearly impossible.

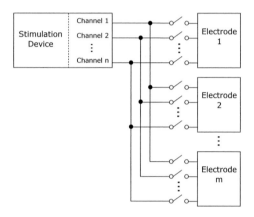

Fig. 5.3. Stimulation channels 1 to n are connected to m electrodes. Type I demultiplexers require n x m switches for multi-channel operation.

5.2 Standalone System for Array Electrode FES

In the scope of this research project a type I demultiplexer was developed at the Institute of Nano- and Medical Electronics of the Hamburg University of Technology. The development process of this system, from now on called Switchbox I, has been described in detail in the Master thesis 'Design einer Multiplexer-Schaltung zur selektiven funktionellen Elektrostimulation' by Ann-Kristin Neumann. A presentation of the system was also published [82] and presented at the 'Dreiländertagung' of the Swiss, Austrian and German societies for biomedical engineering 2016 in Basel.

Switchbox I supports 16 active electrodes for one stimulation channel. Four flex sensors can be connected to determine the most efficient stimulation sites by monitoring finger movements. Switchbox I can be controlled completely with buttons and a keypad. All necessary information are given to the user on a liquid-crystal display.

The complete system (Figure 5.4) consists of a stimulation device, Switchbox I, an array electrode and optional flex sensors. The idea was to design a system that can be operated easily without a PC to provide a robust method to investigate the possibilities of array electrodes.

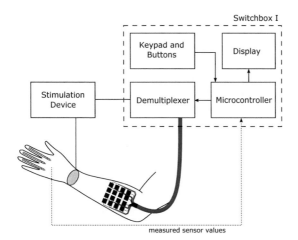

Fig. 5.4. System overview.

5.2.1 Switchbox I

Core of Switchbox I is a microcontroller board (AT91SAM3X8E [83], Arduino Due [84]). The system can be programmed and powered over a micro USB port. An input/output (I/O) expander (MAX7301 [85]) is connected over a Serial Peripheral Interface (SPI) to the microcontroller (Figure 5.5). The output pins of the I/O expander are connected over Darlington transistors to the switches. Reed relays are used as switches and are connected in series to the active electrodes. Since Switchbox I is an example of a type I demultiplexer no information about stimulation pulse timings are available. Therefore, Switchbox I has to be able to prevent current reaching the patient. The used relays can withstand high voltages and currents, offering a complete separation of the patient and the stimulation device. The Darlington transistors are used to offer the necessary current to switch the relays.

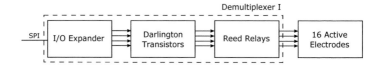

Fig. 5.5. The demultiplexer used in Switchbox I consists of an I/O expander, Darlington transistors and reed relays. 16 active electrodes can be activated with Switchbox I.

To control Switchbox I a 4x4 keypad and two buttons are used. A display allows the user to navigate through different stimulation protocols. Up to four flex sensors can be attached to Switchbox I to measure finger movements over a simple voltage divider. It is possible to control Switchbox I over a serial USB interface. Additionally, sensor values can be monitored more accurately with a connected PC. For normal operation, however, a PC is not necessary.

5.2.2 Stimulation Protocols

As explained in Section 4.3.1 a search function is very useful when using array electrodes for FES. Switchbox I features a search function, automatically determining the desired active electrode. This protocol activates single stimulation electrodes successively and measures finger movement with up to four flex sensors. The two electrodes eliciting the greatest range of motion will be displayed for each flex sensor after the finished search protocol. Stimulation protocols should not be used until an appropriate electrode selection has been performed. Three stimulation protocols were realized for Switchbox I: First, a classical stimulation protocol using one active electrode, second, a protocol activating two electrodes simultaneously for a simple virtual electrode and third DLFS with two electrodes. To perform DLFS two relays are switched with a frequency matching the stimulation frequency.

5.2.3 Conclusion

The here presented stimulation system is a rather simple prototype to perform NMES or FES with array electrodes comparable to systems described in [80] and [81]. It provides a straight forward approach which is easy to use and allows fast stimulation set ups. Switchbox I was designed as an example of a type I demultiplexer and to gather first experiences with array electrodes. Since only one stimulation channel is supported complex stimulation patterns cannot be achieved. The size of Switchbox I prohibits mobile applications. The necessity to control the stimulation device as well as Switchbox I individually makes the handling difficult if changes in stimulation parameters and electrode selection shall be performed at the same time. To allow better handling and more complex stimulation patterns a synchronized demultiplexer should be developed.

5.3 Type II Demultiplexer

Type II demultiplexers offer more direct control of the array electrode. To achieve this they have to be synchronized with the stimulation device. A synchronization offers the possibility of a compact system design and simultaneous control of the stimulation device as well as the demultiplexer, thus, making the handling more intuitive and user friendly. A type II demultiplexer has to be regarded as an extension of a specific stimulation device, whereas a type I demultiplexer can be used with any device.

When demultiplexer and stimulation device are synchronized and the timing of pulses is known it is possible to achieve a multi-channel stimulation without increasing the number of switches. Output from multiple stimulation channels have to be merged for this purpose (Figure 5.6). One merged channel results by shorting multiple output channels or by a using a specific mode of operation. This mode of operation has to be able to output stimulation pulses with different parameters at precisely determined times out of one common output. A special configuration of the MOTIONSTIM 8 (MEDEL GmbH, Hamburg, Germany) stimulation device allows to deliver stimulation pulses in a rapid manner out of one stimulation channel without shorting the channels.

Each stimulation pulse occurs in a known time frame T_{stim}. Closing switches during that time frame will pass the stimulation pulse to the associated electrode on the array. Distributing components of the merged channel to electrodes on the array forms virtual channels (Figure 5.7). Stimulation pulses can also be passed to multiple electrodes at the same time to form virtual electrodes (Section 4.3.2) or to multiple electrodes successively to perform DLFS (Section 4.3.3). Using multiple virtual channels can result in a high number of pulses per second. Since all virtual channels share one output a high number of pulses can occur at the indifferent electrode, unless it is demultiplexed as well. As a consequence attention should be given to that matter to avoid increased stress for the patient. Sharing one indifferent electrode between multiple virtual channels can be beneficial when not many places for appropriate electrode placement are available and the number of pulses per second is manageable. It eases the process of electrode placement and more space on the skin can be left untouched or covered with potential active electrodes.

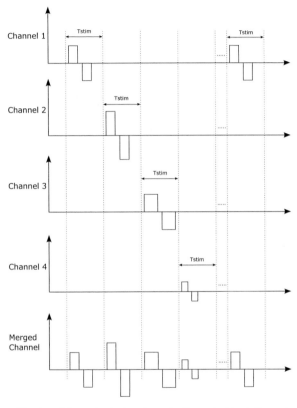

Fig. 5.6. Merging of four stimulation channels. For each stimulation pulse a certain time frame T_{stim} is reserved. Stimulation channels can be shorted to create a merged channel or a programmable stimulation pulse source can be used to output stimulation pulses with different parameters at specific times.

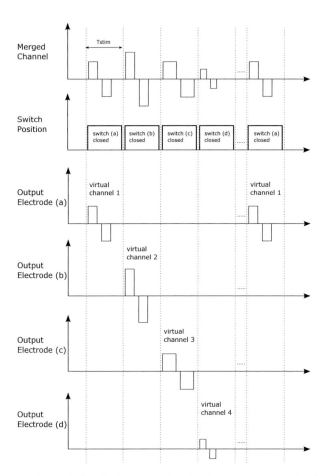

Fig. 5.7. A type II demultiplexer is used to distribute stimulation pulses from the merged channel to designated electrodes forming virtual channels. Precise timings allow switches to act exactly in the correct time frame T_{stim}.

5.4 Fully Synchronized System for Array Electrode FES

As a successor to Switchbox I a new demultiplexer called Switchbox II was designed. A detailed description of the development process can be found in the Master Thesis 'Entwicklung einer drahtlosen Steuerung von Multi-Pad-Elektrostimulation' by Nils Remer. In contrast to Switchbox I described in Section 5.2, Switchbox II does not contain a microcontroller or control elements like buttons or a display. An adapter (Smartstim adapter) is used to control the stimulation unit as well as Switchbox II over Bluetooth. Controlling both devices with a smartphone or tablet allows versatile and mobile applications. The MOTIONSTIM 8 (MEDEL GmbH, Hamburg, Germany) is the stimulation device used for the realization of this type II demultiplexer. A special mode of operation called ScienceMode is utilized to enable a synchronized system.

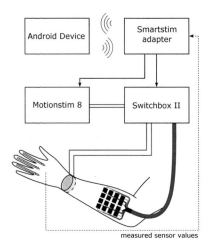

Fig. 5.8. System overview.

Currently Switchbox II supports 32 active and two indifferent electrodes for 8 virtual channels. Four flex sensors can be connected to the Smartstim adapter to determine the most efficient stimulation sites. The MOTIONSTIM 8 and Switchbox II are controlled with an Android application running on a smartphone or tablet.

The complete system (Figure 5.8) consists of an Android device, the MOTIONSTIM 8, the Smartstim adapter, Switchbox II, one or two array electrodes and if desired flex sensors.

5.4.1 MOTIONSTIM 8

The MOTIONSTIM 8 is a certified and available 8-channel stimulation device developed by the company MEDEL GmbH (MEDEL). The outputs are biphasic rectangular stimulation pulses with a $100\,\mu s$ interphase. Stimulation amplitude can be adjusted from 0 to $127\,mA$ in $1\,mA$ steps. The pulse width has a range from 10 to $500\,\mu s$ with a $1\,\mu s$ resolution. Stimulation frequency can be set for each channel individually between 1 and $100\,Hz$.

Four digital switches can be used to trigger certain stimulation events previously programmed with the MOTIONSOFT software. Over a RJ45 connection the MOTION-STIM 8 can be controlled with an external device over a RS232 interface when the ScienceMode is used.

ScienceMode

Information and documents about the ScienceMode were supplied by MEDEL during the scope of the BMBF-project ESiMED. The ScienceMode was originally intended to enable a complete device control over a PC. Two stimulation strategies are available:

- Single Pulse Mode

- Channel List Mode

Single Pulse Mode A single command send to the MOTIONSTIM 8 will cause one stimulation pulse immediately after the command has been processed. The command contains all the information about the stimulation pulse including channel number, amplitude and pulse width. Sending multiple commands to the MOTIONSTIM 8 can generate complex patterns. The timing of the stimulation pulses, hence, the stimulation frequency, is completely controlled by the external device. Commands send at a high frequency will cause a high frequency stimulation. Also the timings between pulses from different channels need to be determined by the external device. Thus, controlling the MOTIONSTIM 8 over the Single Pulse Mode with a PC is quite challenging.

The operation system of the PC makes it difficult to send commands with a constant frequency at accurate timings. However, a microcontroller connected to the MOTIONSTIM 8 can achieve very accurate timings, making the Single Pulse Mode the optimal method to control the MOTIONSTIM 8 with complete control over every stimulation pulse.

Channel List Mode To simplify the generation of complex stimulation patterns and to allow a robust control with a PC the Channel List Mode exists. In this mode the MOTIONSTIM 8 is responsible for the stimulation pulse timings. The received commands will start a train of stimulation pulses with the desired parameters at the desired channel.

Since the stimulation pulse timings can be precisely controlled with a microcontroller the Single Pulse Mode is the utilized mode of operation.

5.4.2 Smartstim Adapter

As previously explained the utility of the ScienceMode can be enhanced considerably with an external microcontroller by using the Single Pulse Mode in its full potential. The microcontroller has two main tasks: First, to determine the timing of stimulation pulses and to select the desired electrodes. Second, to enable wireless bidirectional communication with another device, e.g. a smartphone.

There are two main components on the Smartstim adapter (Figure 5.9). A microcontroller (ATmega328 [86]) and a Bluetooth Low Energy (BLE) chip (CC2540 [87]). Both are located on a Bluno Nano [88] board from DFRobot. Additionally, a level shifter, to generate RS232 signals the MOTIONSTIM 8 can process, and a resistor network to form voltage dividers for flex sensors are used. The Smartstim adapter is powered directly by the 8.2 V output of the MOTIONSTIM 8. The microcontroller handles two serial connections, one to the MOTIONSTIM 8 and a wireless one (enabled by the BLE chip) to the Android device.

5.4.3 Switchbox II

Switchbox II can only be operated in conjunction with the Smartstim adapter and the MOTIONSTIM 8. Since the Smartstim adapter is doing all the processing and communication Switchbox II could be realized as minimalistic system (Figure 5.10). It is

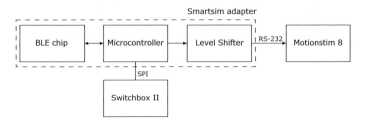

Fig. 5.9. The smartstim adapter communicates over Bluetooth Low Energy (BLE) with an Android device. The level shifter transforms commands from the microcontroller into RS-232 signals for the MOTIONSTIM 8. The microcontroller communicates over a Serial Peripheral Interface (SPI) with Switchbox II.

a stackable system consisting of a I/O expander (MAX6957 [89]) and MOSFET relays (G3VM-351G [90]). The I/O expander is connected over a SPI with the microcontroller on the Smartstim adapter. Switchbox II is powered like the Smartstim adapter directly from the MOTIONSTIM 8. The MOSFET relays are connected directly to the I/O expander because the MAX6957 can operate its outputs as adjustable current sinks. Hence, the MOSFET relays can be controlled without series resistances or Darlington transistors. The MOSFET relays offer faster switching times compared to reed relays at the cost of a mechanical separation. They still are capable to withstand up to 110 mA and 350 V. Section 5.4.4 will explain that due to the synchronized operation of the stimulation device and the demultiplexer the MOSFET relays do not have to prevent current reaching the patient, even though they could do it.

The boards of Switchbox II are stackable enabling 16 active electrodes per board. Four boards could be stacked to reach 64 electrodes. Each board does also contain outputs and switches for two indifferent electrodes. Currently the Smartstim adapter is only programmed for stimulation with up to 32 active and two indifferent electrodes. Switchbox II contains an input that can be used to connect a device for biosignal acquisition. Some additional switches were designated for the purpose of EMG measurements through the electrode array.

5.4.4 Stimulation Pulse Timing and Electrode Selection

To achieve a reliable timing and correct distribution to elements on the array electrode for each stimulation pulse, independent of its duration, a certain time frame is reserved.

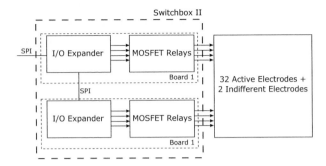

Fig. 5.10. Two stacked boards form Switchbox II. Both boards are identical and have an I/O expander and multiple MOSFET relays. The I/O expanders are controlled over a Serial Peripheral Interface (SPI). 32 active and 2 indifferent electrodes can be activated by Switchbox II.

During this time frame a specific sequence of events is initiated forming a stimulation frame. One stimulation frame has the following structure:

1. Begin of Stimulation Frame: Command to close associated switches

2. 1 ms later: Command to trigger a stimulation pulse

3. 2 ms later: Command to open associated switches again

4. 1 ms later: End of stimulation frame

The total duration of one stimulation frame is 4 ms. 1 ms is reserved to ensure the desired switches are closed before the stimulation pulse is generated. The time between closing and opening of the switches is 2 ms. The maximum duration of one biphasic stimulation pulse is 1.1 ms (two 500 μs pulses with a 100 μs interphase), thus giving the MOTIONSTIM 8 enough time to process the stimulation command and to generate the pulse. The stimulation frame is terminated 1 ms after the command to close the switches to ensure no switches are closed when the next stimulation frame starts. The timings during one stimulation frame are chosen conservatively to warrant predictable and safe stimulation conditions.

The complete stimulation process is designed in a loop. The stimulation frequency determines the duration of one loop iteration. One loop contains eight stimulation frames corresponding to eight virtual channels. The events of one stimulation frame will only occur when the corresponding virtual channel is set to active. Otherwise no events take place, meaning switches are not closed and opened and no stimulation command is sent to the MOTIONSTIM 8. After all stimulation frames the loop will wait to match the desired stimulation frequency. With eight virtual channels one loop lasts at least 32 ms. Therefore, the maximum stimulation frequency is limited to about 30 Hz. It is possible to use higher stimulation frequencies by reducing the number of allowed virtual channels.

5.4.5 System Control

The whole System is controlled wirelessly with an external Android device. The microcontroller is handling the communication to the Android device. A special communication protocol was developed to allow complete control of the system with external devices, in this case Android smartphones or tablets. The communication protocol could also be used to connect a PC or laptop via USB or wirelessly. There is a list of commands used to control the complete stimulation system. Commands can be divided into the following categories:

- Pulse Parameter Settings

- Channel Activation and Stimulation Status

- Electrode Selection

- Information Exchange and Safety Features

Pulse Parameter Settings

Settings like amplitude, pulse width and frequency can be controlled comfortably over the Android device. Amplitude and pulse width can be set for each channel individually, whereas, stimulation frequency is global for all virtual channels. At the end of one iteration of the stimulation loop all these parameters can be updated. The updated parameters are then used for the next iteration, allowing a pulse by pulse control.

Channel Activation and Stimulation Status

In order to perform a stimulation the desired virtual channels have to be activated and the stimulation status has to be set to on. Otherwise the stimulation loop will not be executed. Stimulation on single channels can be terminated by deactivating the corresponding virtual channel and be activated vice versa. Stimulation on all active channels can be stopped by changing the stimulation status to off. The stimulation status and channel activation is checked and updated at the end of every stimulation loop iteration.

Electrode Selection

For each virtual channel up to four active electrodes can be selected for simultaneously or successively activation. Comparable to the pulse parameter settings, the electrode selection can be changed at the end of each iteration of a stimulation loop. Different virtual channels are not allowed to share electrodes. The user can decide to use two indifferent electrodes.

Information Exchange and Safety Features

It is important for the user to know which settings are currently used in operation. Hence, a bidirectional communication is necessary. Commands send from the Android device to the stimulation system are confirmed by the Smartstim adapter. This way the Android device can visualize the currently used settings for the user. A change in settings will only be completed if a confirmation is received.

Additionally, the stimulation system needs to know whether the Android control device is still connected and operating properly. Therefore, a refresh signal is send regularly from the Android device to the Smartstim adapter during stimulation. If the Smartstim adapter does not receive a refresh signal for a defined time the stimulation will be terminated.

5.4.6 Stimulation Protocols

Similar to the system described in Section 5.2 a search function can be performed. Four flex sensors can be connected to the Smartstim adapter. The electrode search function will be started with the Android device. Due to the higher resolution of the Android device compared to the display of Switchbox I the four electrodes that measure the greatest finger extension are displayed for each sensor.

Stimulation can be performed with eight independent channels. Every of these virtual channels can have its own stimulation parameters and set of electrodes. For each channel a maximum of four electrodes can be selected for simultaneous or successive activation. During successive activation the active electrode will be changed for every stimulation loop iteration, hence performing DLFS. Stimulation protocols can be configured for each channel individually. It is possible to use DLFS on some channels, form virtual electrodes of two, three or four elements on other channels and to do simple one electrode stimulation on the remaining channels.

Since all the virtual channels are generated from one stimulation output they share an indifferent electrode. In case of many active channels the number of pulses per second can be high. Hence, it is possible to activate two indifferent electrodes successively to avoid discomfort due to high frequency stimulation beneath a single indifferent electrode.

5.4.7 Conclusion

The here presented systems demonstrates a distinct advance compared to the system described in Section 5.2. A more compact design, eight independent stimulation channels with 32 active and two indifferent electrodes together with a intuitive wireless control were achieved. This system enables the complete exploitation of array electrodes and a transfer in real-life applications.

This performance comes with the cost of being dependent on the MOTIONSTIM 8. A more compact stimulation unit would be preferable and is something to work on in the future. The possibility to use individual stimulation frequencies for each stimulation channel was lost with the realization of stimulation pulse timings on the Smartstim adapter. Completely adjustable frequencies for each channel would exacerbate safe and reliable electrode selection greatly and was therefore sacrificed. It is however possible to reduce stimulation frequencies for individual channels by skipping stimulation loop iterations, albeit, this function is not yet realized.

5.5 System Comparison

In this section a comparison of the system introduced in Section 5.4 to similar systems presented in other studies will be described. An overview of systems offering the possibility to perform FES with array electrodes was given in [70]. Here, a selection of these systems and some systems that were not mentioned in [70] are listed in Table 5.1.

Especially the number of supported electrodes, the channel count, wireless support and wearability are considered of great importance. All systems listed in Table 5.1 with the exception of Kenney et al. [72] are designed with stimulation of the upper extremities in mind. The ShefStim stimulation system is designed for drop foot applications. All systems support at least 32 electrodes, thereby providing a sufficient amount of stimulation sites for most stimulation scenarios. Very high electrode numbers may require a long set up to find appropriate electrode configurations or demand the formation of virtual electrodes. Multi-channel stimulation is required if different movements shall be performed or combined at will. The systems from Lawrence et al. [91] and Exell et al. [81] enable stimulation with 4 channels, at the cost of wearability due to big demultiplexer hardware.

The INTFES [7] and INTFES v2 [92] are stimulation devices, specifically designed for FES with array electrodes and have been used in numerous publications [65, 64, 7, 69, 92]. Even though the INTFES devices are described as 1 channel stimulators, they can form stimulation patterns combined out of several pulses with distinctive properties, timings and associated electrodes.

The first system from Valtin et al. [93] is based on an 8 channel stimulator, hence potentially allowing multi-channel applications. However, each channel requires an own demultiplexer, resulting in an overall bulky system. The new system from Valtin et al. [94] based on the RehaMovePro seems to be a distinct improvement to their previous development. It is however unclear how many channels can be switched by one demultiplexer. The high maximum stimulation frequency of 500 Hz could indicate that virtual stimulation channels may be formed, similar to the system introduced in this thesis (Section 5.4). Both systems from Valtin et al. provide synchronization between the stimulation device and the demultiplexer which they use to measure muscle activity in form of an EMG between stimulation pulses.

For mobile applications and to incorporate sensor data from external systems a wireless interface is used in [7, 92, 94] and Section 5.4. Wearable solutions and wireless interfaces are especially important to support patients that still maintain some mobility, such as many stroke survivors. Treatment of patients who are suffering from a SCI and are depending on a wheelchair has a smaller need for mobile and wearable stimulation systems.

The system developed in the scope of this thesis is the only wearable full synchronized system that is based on a commercially available and certified stimulation device, making it suited for future clinical studies and applications. Furthermore, the modular structure and the synchronization method can be used as a model for a future stimulation device development.

Tab. 5.1. Comparison of systems for electrical stimulation with array electrodes.

	Lawrence et al. [91]	Exell et al. [81]	Malesevic et al. [7]	Malesevic et al. [92]	Kenney et al. [72]	Valtin et al. [93]	Valtin et al. [94]	Loitz et al. Section 5.4
Stimulator	Compex Motion 2 [95]	INTFES (not commercially available)	INTFES v2 (not commercially available)	Modified Oddstock stimulator	ShefStim (not commercially available)	RehaMove	Reha-MovePro (not commercially available)	MOTION-STIM 8
Electrodes	256 (active or indif.)	32 active, 1 indif.	32 active, 1 indif.	64 active, 1 indif.	64 active, 1 indif.	60 active, 4 indif.	48 active, 2 indif., 11 flexible	32 active, 2 indif.
Channels	4	4	1	1	64	1	4	8
Control	PC	PC	PC	PC	PC	PC	tablet/PC	Android device
Wireless	no	yes	yes	no	no	no	yes	yes
Wearable	no	yes	yes	no	yes	no	yes	yes

6 Sensor based Stimulation Control

It is the goal to increase the quality of life for persons affected by neuronal impairments with FES techniques that are included in real-life applications. Therefore, intuitive methods to trigger stimulations are necessary. Switches or sensor systems can be used to generate control signals that start or stop specific stimulation patterns. Feedback controlled stimulation can increase the effectiveness of FES and simplify the process. Section 6.1 will give an overview of possible methods for stimulation device control. A wireless adjustable system to control FES applications will be introduced in Section 6.2. Sensors can not only be used to start and stop stimulation patterns, they can also provide feedback of the stimulation effect to the system. This feedback can then be used to adjust stimulation settings accordingly, e.g. controlling stimulation intensity. Section 6.3 will describe two feedback based approaches for intensity control.

6.1 Stimulation Device Control

Most home applications of FES or NMES are done with pre-programmed stimulation devices [5] where stimulation parameters are set and the therapy is performed passively for a set duration without active intervention of the subject. Techniques like stimulation assisted mirror therapy [13, 14, 16] or biofeedback controlled stimulation [3] are aiming in an active participation during the training sessions for an increased training and relearning effect. For this purpose mechanical data or muscle activity are measured and used to trigger stimulation events.

Especially FES applications, trying to achieve coordinated movements that can be used to improve the daily quality of life for patients who suffer from a SCI or stroke, often require active methods to trigger or even control electrical stimulation.

6.1.1 Sensors and Switches used to Trigger Stimulation Events

Several kinds of mechanical switches or sensors have been used to trigger or control electrical stimulation. One of the most widely known example is the treatment of foot drop caused by stroke with electrical stimulation of the peroneal nerve in the leg [5]. To correct foot drop a heel switch or pressure sensor is placed in the shoe and used to trigger and stop the stimulation. In a systematic review Kottink et al. showed that the usage of FES results in an increased walking speed for impaired patients [96].

Stimulation of the upper extremities, e.g. for grasping neuroprosthesis, can be controlled with several kinds of sensors or switches. Popovic et al. offered patients suffering from SCI the possibility to control a grasping neuroprosthesis with a push button or sliding potentiometer [6].

Rupp et al. [8] used a shoulder joystick to achieve lateral grasp and palmar grasp patterns with a surface electrode based neuroprosthesis. The control of the system with a shoulder joystick and the achieved grasping patterns are comparable to the Freehand system [12].

Stimulation control with the tongue is technically possible but not well accepted by patients because of cosmetic reasons and the negative impact on communication [97].

6.1.2 Electromyography Triggered Stimulation

EMG-triggered FES is a technique used to facilitate recovery after stroke. The remaining muscle functions of the impaired limb are used to trigger a stimulation event that elicits the lost movement. The patient is required to contract muscle fibers that are involved in the desired movement in order to generate an electric signal that can be amplified and processed. Once the EMG signal strength surpasses a threshold a stimulation is initialized for a pre-defined duration that will lead to the movement the subject tried to perform. An enhancement in voluntary motor control due to EMG-triggered FES was reported in [98] and [99].

During EMG-triggered FES in most cases the same electrodes are used for measuring muscle activity and performing electrical stimulation. Using the same electrodes for stimulation and measuring of muscle activity requires a separation of the measuring circuit from the electrodes during stimulation. Therefore, commercial systems like the STIWELL med4 [100](MED-EL GmbH, Innsbruck, Austria) or Mentastim [101](TQ-

Systems GmbH, Seefeld, Germany) have a pre-defined duration of the stimulation phase. In these cases the EMG signal is only used to turn on the stimulation, not to turn it off. A disadvantage of this technique is that due to the predefined stimulation durations it is difficult to perform functional task-oriented training, like grasping and moving an object. It is also only possible to detect the intention of movement before the stimulation phase begins, once the stimulation has started there is no way to ensure the movement intention is still present.

6.1.3 Brain-Computer Interface

A brain-computer interface allows scientists to form a direct communication from the brain to a computer [102]. The electric signal in the motor cortex produced by brain activity can be measured with surface electrodes. These electrodes are typically included in a cap and cover most parts of the scalp. These recorded brain patters are referred to as an electroencephalogram (EEG).

Rohm et al. used a hybrid BCI system to control a hybrid FES based neuroprosthesis for an individual suffering from SCI [11]. The hybrid BCI consists of the EEG-recording system and a shoulder joystick. The hybrid neuroprosthesis includes the FES system, responsible for grasping functions, and a mechanical orthesis to enable elbow movements.

In a recent project Bouton et al. used an implanted intracortical microelectrode array to measure the brain activity of an individual suffering from SCI [103]. The decoded brain activity was used to control an electrode array based FES system, allowing the subject to perform distinct hand and finger movements.

Using a BCI efficiently requires a lot of training and a time consuming set up. There are not many other options for severely impaired patients to regain some independence and quality of life. Patients with a hemiplegia due to stroke still maintain some mobility which would be affected negatively by a BCI. Furthermore, cosmetic reasons make a high acceptance of BCI systems including an EEG cap unlikely.

6.2 FES Control with Wireless Sensor Systems

The severity of hand impairment of stroke survivors can vary to a great extent, leaving some individuals with a limited range of motion, whereas others suffer from a complete loss of functionality. Mobile and customizable systems can help these patients to obtain an adequate training option or an intuitively controlled neuroprosthesis for everyday life activities. Here, an extension of the system presented in Section 5.4 will be introduced.

6.2.1 Principle

The addition of sensors into a neuroprosthesis is nothing new. Sensor data can be used to start and stop stimulation events or to determine stimulation intensity. The system described in Section 5.4 offers a wireless BLE interface. A smartphone or tablet is able to maintain several Bluetooth connections at the same time. Sensor data obtained by another external system can be evaluated by the Android device and used for FES control (Figure 6.1). Including sensors wirelessly with another component instead of connecting them directly to the Smartstim adapter has the advantage that the firmware on the adapter does not have to be modified. The firmware on the Smartstim adapter includes the complete state machine for the pulse timings, persons not familiar with the whole system could potentially make changes that affect the functionality and safety of the system. In this modular approach sensor values can easily be sent to the android device and evaluated there to generate the corresponding commands for the Smartstim adapter.

6.2.2 Flex Sensor Triggered Stimulation

Flex sensors are an easy method to measure and evaluate finger movements and therefore particularly suited for the determination of efficient stimulation sites on an array electrode (Section 4.3.1). Here, they are used to generate trigger signals for the stimulation device when an adjustable threshold is surpassed. Stimulation persists until the sensor value drops below the threshold. Possible locations of flex sensors for trigger generation are fingers of the impaired hand, the wrist or the fingers of the healthy contralateral hand. Using flex sensors on fingers of the impaired hand can recognize small movements that correspond to the intention of hand opening. Fingers of the impaired

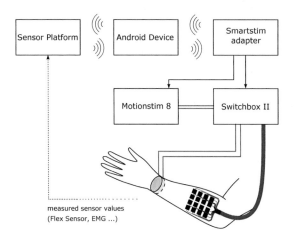

Fig. 6.1. System overview. An additional device to acquire sensor data can be connected to the Android device.

hand can also be opened by the healthy hand to trigger a stimulation event. A still preserved mobility of the wrist can be assessed with flex sensors as well. An extension or flexion of the wrist can be interpreted as a trigger for a certain grasping pattern. A contralateral control can be achieved with flex sensors attached to the fingers of the healthy hand, enabling the impaired hand to mimic movements of the healthy one. Flex sensors can be exchanged easily for different sensors, e.g. pressure sensors for applications on the lower limps, or acceleration sensors to measure rotations of the wrist.

6.2.3 Electromyography Controlled Stimulation

Utilizing the remaining muscle activity of impaired patients to control a grasping neuroprosthesis can result in an intuitive system adequate for daily life applications [97]. The EMG signal can be used as a switch to turn stimulations on or off or even to grade the stimulation intensity [6].

Stimulation pulses during FES have a large amplitude compared to the EMG signal generated by voluntary muscle contractions. Therefore, measuring electrodes have to be placed with some distance to the stimulation electrodes. This can be especially challenging when array electrodes are used that cover a large portion of the stimulated muscles. At the Institute of Nano- and Medical Electronics of the Hamburg University of Technology a platform for biosignal acquisition based on a ATSAM3X8E microcontroller [83] and an 8-channel 24 bit analog-to-digital converter from Texas Instruments (ADS1299 [104]) was developed. A detailed description of this system can be found in the Master thesis 'Development of a modular and mobile platform for biopotential detection and control signal generation' by Till Sellschopp. The biosignal acquisition platform contains a Bluetooth module, enabling it to send sensor values to an Android application.

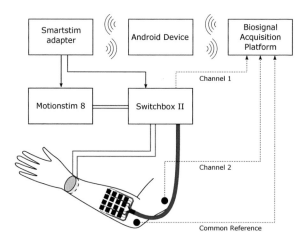

Fig. 6.2. Overview of the stimulation system extended by a biosignal acquisition platform. The muscle activity of the forearm and upper arm are used to start and stop stimulation events.

The EMG controlled stimulation shall detect the intention of the subject to open the hand. When electrode arrays are used for the stimulation they cover the area that could be used for the EMG recording. Thus, the EMG has to be measured through the electrode array. To protect the recording hardware no EMG can be measured as long as the stimulation lasts. Voluntary contractions of the extensor muscles in the forearm are typically accompanied by contractions of muscles in the upper arm (cocontractions). The idea is to use these contractions, or rather the lack of them, to decide when the stimulation shall stop. Therefore, one channel is connected to the electrode array through switchbox II, the other channel is placed on the upper arm, e.g. the triceps brachii muscle (Figure 6.2). The EMG signal of both channels has to surpass an individual threshold to trigger the stimulation. Once the stimulation is activated the switches connecting the biosignal platform to the electrode array are opened, leaving the input of this channel floating. Hence, this channel cannot record any evaluable data during the stimulation. The second channel on the upper arm is still recording and used to decide how long the stimulation shall persist. As soon as the EMG signal of the upper arm channel falls below the threshold the stimulation is stopped. At this point the switches connecting the MOTIONSTIM 8 to the electrode array open and the switches connecting the biosignal acquisition platform to the array close, hence, enabling EMG recordings on both channels. These recordings can then again be used to trigger a new stimulation. This technique constitutes a distinct enhancement compared to classical EMG-triggered stimulation as training method. Due to the measurement of cocontractions during the stimulation phase is is possible to detect whether the subject wants the stimulation to continue or to stop, making the control way more direct and natural.

6.2.4 Conclusion

The possibilities for FES applications provided by sensor data acquired by a wireless device connected over Bluetooth to an Android device are nearly limitless. The here presented approach is the foundation for individualized FES systems that can be adjusted to the patient depending on his condition and needs. Combinations of mechanical sensors like flex sensors and EMG signals are just one possibility that can now easily be realized. Clinical trials are now necessary to develop a set of sensors and switches that achieve a high acceptance and can then finally lead to systems that allow a comfortable and intuitive integration in daily life activities or to enable natural and motivating training techniques.

6.3 Feedback Controlled Stimulation

Finding correct stimulation parameters can be a challenging task for a therapist and especially for an impaired patient at home. The effect of stimulation parameters can also change during a FES or NMES application. One possible reason is neuromuscular fatigue but also changes in the electrode skin contact might require an adjustment of the stimulation intensity. During a short training session this might not be a big problem, but systems that are supposed to support the patient in daily life activities are absolutely dependent on appropriate stimulation parameters.

Here, two approaches of feedback based pulse intensity control are presented.

6.3.1 Simple Smart Pulse Intensity Control

Closed-loop FES systems, using sensor feedback for adjustments of stimulation parameters, typically include software running on a connected PC. Here, a simple approach of a closed-loop intensity control, running completely on an external microcontroller, will be explained. This approach was published [105] and presented at the 'Dreiländertagung' of the Swiss, Austrian and German societies for biomedical engineering 2016 in Basel. The system uses a commercial stimulation unit that is programmable and has multiple digital inputs. For the intensity control a microcontroller board is connected to the digital inputs of the MOTIONSTIM 8 (Figure 6.3). In order to evaluate finger movement flex sensors are attached to the hand of the subject and connected to the microcontroller board using a voltage divider. With these sensors even small changes in the position of the fingers can be detected.

Figure 6.4 shows the general principle of the intensity control. The idea is to increase the stimulation intensity stepwise until an efficient hand opening is achieved. When the stimulation intensity is increased in small steps the hand will start to open. Until a certain movement threshold is surpassed the intensity will be increased to leave the subthreshold intensity range. When an intensity increase leads to a meaningful change of the finger movement this intensity increase is regarded as efficient and the intensity will be increased even further. At some point an increase in stimulation intensity will not result in a further opening of the hand, this is the point when the increase of stimulation intensity has become inefficient. Inefficient increases will be undone and the stimulation intensity will stay at the previous level. This level of intensity is then regarded as the optimal stimulation intensity. The stimulation will then continue with this intensity until it is terminated by the user or the intensity becomes insufficient to keep the hand open due to muscle fatigue. If the hand opening decreases the intensity

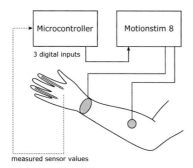

Fig. 6.3. An external microcontroller board is connected to the digital inputs of the MOTIONSTIM 8. Three digital inputs are used to perform the intensity control.

control will react and increase the intensity again, trying to restore the original finger position.

The intensity control is realized with two state machines, one on the microcontroller and one directly programmed on the MOTIONSTIM 8. The program on the MOTION-STIM 8 was generated using a tool called MOTIONSOFT (MEDEL GmbH, Hamburg, Germany) and is interpreting digital signals from the microcontroller to set the correct stimulation intensity. The actual intensity control runs on the microcontroller and is responsible to measure and evaluate sensor data as well as to send the corresponding commands to the MOTIONSTIM 8.

MOTIONSTIM Program

The MOTIONSTIM 8 provides four digital inputs that can be used to enter and leave up to 30 programmed stimulation states. The intensity control presented here requires three digital inputs and uses all available stimulation states. Digital input 1 is used to start the stimulation. As long as input 1 receives a low signal the stimulation continues. Input 2 is responsible to decrease stimulation intensity. Receiving a low signal will decrease stimulation intensity. Input 3 handles the intensity increases. A low signal at input 3 will result in a jump to the next intensity level. The MOTIONSTIM 8 prioritizes low number inputs over higher number inputs. Thus, input 1 has the highest

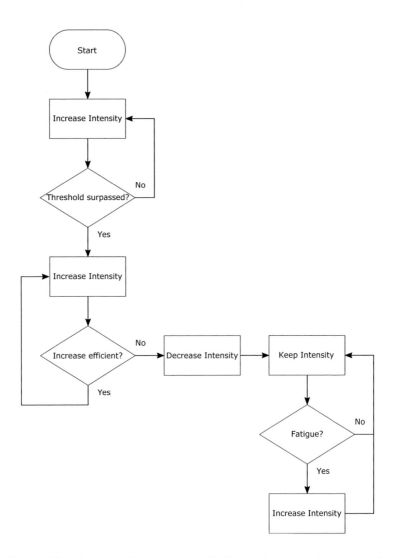

Fig. 6.4. Flow diagram of the intensity control. The stimulation intensity is increased until a threshold value of the flex sensor is surpassed and then until a increase of the stimulation intensity did not lead to a meaningful change of the sensor value (Increase efficient? - no). Then the intensity is decreased once and kept on that level until the sensor value starts to drop which indicates fatigue. The stimulation can be terminated at any point by the user.

priority and is therefore responsible to start and stop the stimulation. The intensity levels were realized by varying the pulse widths. The stimulation amplitude has to be set manually on the stimulation device.

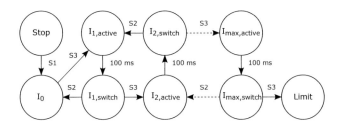

Fig. 6.5. State machine on the MOTIONSTIM 8. Signals to the digital inputs 1, 2 and 3 (S1, S2 and S3) are used to move from one intensity level to another. To simplify matters connections to the state *stop* were not illustrated. When S1 turns high the program will move to *stop* from every state.

Figure 6.5 illustrates the structure of the MOTIONSTIM state machine. The program starts at the state *stop*. A low signal to input 1 will result in a jump to the first intensity level I_0. If no low signal is received at input 1 during the stimulation state will move to the stop state immediately. A low signal at input 3 will cause the stimulation state to move to the next intensity level I_1. Starting from I_1 all intensity levels consist of two states. One active state $I_{i,active}$ and one switching state $I_{i,switch}$. The program will enter the active state after every change in stimulation for 100 ms. The active state prevents the program to perform jumps over multiple intensity levels. After 100 ms the program moves to the switching state. From there the intensity can be lowered with a low signal at input 2 or increased again with a low signal at input 3. This method allows to move through 14 different intensity levels safely (50 µs to 174 µs in 10 % steps). Trying to increase the intensity after reaching the final intensity level $I_{max,switch}$ will move the program to state called *limit*, terminating the stimulation and informing the user that the maximum intensity was reached and no optimal intensity was found. In this case the user has to increase the stimulation amplitude manually on the device before the intensity control is used again.

Due to the limited amount of digital inputs and stimulation states the intensity control could only be achieved for one independent channel. If multiple channels shall be used they would all have to follow the same intensity scheme, or just one of them would include the feedback based intensity control.

Microcontroller Firmware

The microcontroller is sampling the sensor data and applies a median filter. The filtered sensor data is the basis for any decision regarding the stimulation intensity. At the moment just data from one flex sensor is used to achieve the intensity control. A second sensor is still evaluated for visualization purposes. The implementation of the intensity control on the microcontroller is loop based. During one loop iteration three things happen:

1. Collect and filter sensor data

2. Send debug data via USB

3. Check control states

Four control states are used to generate output commands for the MOTIONSTIM 8 (Figure 6.6). The first state is the *idle* state. In this state no stimulation is performed and the output 1 will be kept high. Moreover, the sensor value in this state is collected and used as an adapting starting point to evaluate the degree of hand opening. To leave the idle state a start command from the user is necessary. A stop command will move the control state back to *idle* at any time.

A start command will move the state to *stimulation*. The state *stimulation* turns on the stimulation by setting output 1 to low. Additionally, the finger position is evaluated to decide whether an increase (output 3 = low) or decrease (output 2 = low) shall be performed. There are three reasons why the state can move to *increase*. First, the state will move to *increase* every iteration where the sensor value has not yet surpassed a certain threshold (reason: no reaction). Second, the state will move to *increase* in every iteration where the sensor value has increased in a meaningful way compared to the previous iteration, meaning the increase in stimulation intensity was efficient (reason: efficient increase). Third, the state will move to *increase* when the final sensor value is dropping by a certain amount after the final intensity was found (reason: fatigue).

The state *decrease* will be reached in the loop iteration where no meaningful increase of the sensor value was observed compared to the previous iteration, meaning the last intensity increase was inefficient (reason: inefficient increase).

The states *increase* and *decrease* are only accessed for 10 ms which is just enough time

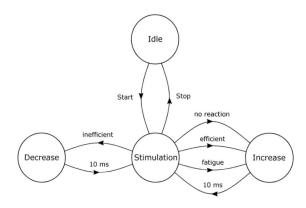

Fig. 6.6. Control states implemented on the microcontroller. The user can start and stop the stimulation manually. Sensor data are used by the intensity control to decide whether states have to move to *increase* or *decrease*.

to allow the MOTIONSTIM 8 to jump from one state to another. After that the state will move back to *stimulation* in order to keep the stimulation running.

The thresholds for 'no reaction', 'efficient increase' and 'fatigue' can be adjusted easily to customize the intensity control.

Start and stop commands are currently provided by the user over USB but could easily be generated by switches or sensors connected to the microcontroller.

A demonstration of the closed-loop intensity control is depicted in Figure 6.7. The feedback controlled stimulation is able to maintain a stable opening of the hand. Figure 6.8 shows how the feedback controlled stimulation reacts to a sudden decrease of finger extension and maintains a complete hand opening by an automatic increase of stimulation intensity.

6.3.2 Calibration based Pulse Intensity Control

Similar to the intensity control described in Section 6.3.1 an intensity control can also be achieved with the wireless sensor system (Section 6.2). The evaluation of sensor values and generation of commands for the stimulation device is performed by a custom written Android application that is based on the results of the Master thesis 'Mobile neurorehabilitation using a modular platform for wireless acquisition of mechanical

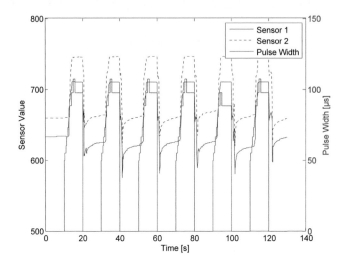

Fig. 6.7. Flex sensor values and stimulation pulse width during successive stimulation with closed-loop intensity control. The hand opening could be maintained on a stable level.

data' by Taylan Ünal. In contrast to the previous approach this intensity control is based on a calibration, performed before the actual stimulation starts. The calibration itself is very similar to the intensity control from Section 6.3.1. The idea is to first surpass a minimum range of motion and then increase the intensity until no meaningful reaction is observed (Figure 6.9).

This calibration works for multiple channels at the same time. Channels can each have a single flex sensor or sensors can be shared among channels. Once a channel is calibrated the stimulation is terminated for this channel and the last efficient intensity is saved as the target intensity and the corresponding sensor value as the target sensor value. The target intensities and sensor values are then used for the stimulation with intensity control.

A flowchart of the calibration based intensity control is depicted in Figure 6.10. The intensity control starts with a stimulation intensity smaller than the target intensity. If the target sensor value of a channel was already reached with this intensity no further increase is performed and the target intensity is reduced. In the next step the

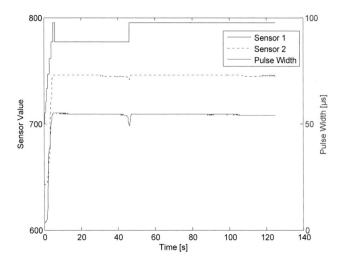

Fig. 6.8. Flex sensor values and stimulation pulse width during continuous stimulation with closed-loop intensity control. A sudden drop of sensor 1 could be balanced out with an automatic pulse width increase.

target intensity is used. If the sensor values do not match the target sensor values the intensity can be increased stepwise until the target sensor value is finally reached. A counter is limiting the number of possible intensity increases above 100 %. Using intensities above 100 % results in an increase of the target intensity for the next stimulation event. The intensity control works for each channel in parallel but independently.

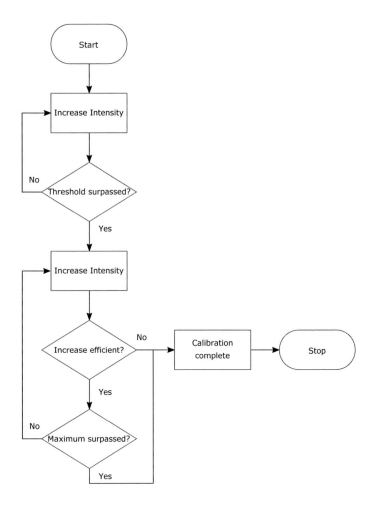

Fig. 6.9. Flow diagram of the intensity calibration. The calibration is performed for multiple stimulation channels at the same time. For each channel the calibration can be completed at different stimulation intensities, depending on the sensor feedback.

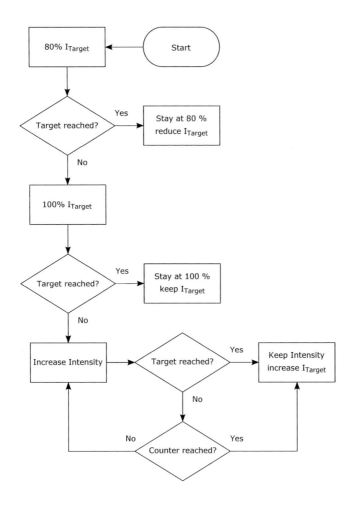

Fig. 6.10. Flow diagram of the calibration based intensity control. The intensity control is performed for multiple stimulation channels at the same time. Each channel can stay at a different stimulation intensity, depending on the sensor feedback. Stimulation can be stopped at any point during the control.

6.3.3 Conclusion

Feedback based intensity control provides a method to counteract neuromuscular fatigue and other reasons altering the necessary stimulation intensity to achieve a specific task. An automatic determination of the stimulation intensity based on a calibration eases the process of self-applied FES tremendously. In the future, sensor feedback can also be used to change the stimulation site on the electrode array, e.g. to react to a rotation of the forearm.

Feedback controlled stimulation in conjunction with a wireless sensor system allows the development of a robust and easy to control neuroprosthesis that can be fitted exactly to the patients' needs. Including the sensors and stimulation electrodes in an unobtrusive orthesis or making the whole system visually appealing is a major task for future applications employing the here presented methods.

7 Experimental Findings

During this project three studies with healthy subjects and stroke survivors were performed. The goals were to assess the effect of NMES in stroke patients, the effectiveness of short stimulation pulses and to demonstrate the efficacy of feedback based intensity control. In the following sections these studies and their results will be presented.

7.1 Decreasing Effect in NMES of Stroke Patients

As already mentioned in Section 2.2.5 increased neuromuscular fatigue is a major challenge in successful applications of electrical stimulation, especially for neuroprotheses. This was demonstrated for healthy controls [106] as well as individuals with SCI [107]. Surprisingly, data demonstrating a reduced fatigue resistance during NMES in stroke survivors is rare, one example is a study of Gerrits et al. reporting increased fatigue during NMES induced knee extension compared to healthy subjects [108]. Stroke survivors often suffer from an extensive spasticity of flexor muscles of the forearm, possibly impeding the effect of NMES even more. Therefore, a study was performed measuring the impact of NMES on force generation and finger extension in a heterogeneous group of stroke survivors. Additionally, the influence of NMES on spasticity was examined.

Here, a short summary of this study which was performed in cooperation with the Department of Neurology of the University Medical Center Hamburg-Eppendorf will be presented. A short version of the study was already published [109] and a full version was submitted for publication.

7.1.1 Methods

Subjects

9 chronic stroke patients (mean time after stroke = 57.9 month +/- 27.6 SD) with a broad spectrum of spasticity and degree of motor impairment (mean age = 55.1 years

+/- 10.8 SD, 3 female) participated in the study. All patients gave written informed consent according to the Declaration of Helsinki. The study was approved by the local ethics committee of the Medical Association of Hamburg (PV4618).

Material

Stimulation Device: The MOTIONSTIM 8 (Section 5.4.1) was used in this study.

Stimulation Electrodes: Pals (Axelgaard, Fallbrook, CA, USA) electrodes were used. The indifferent electrode was elliptic 4 x 6 cm^2, the active electrode round with a 3.2 cm diameter.

Force Gauge: PCE-FG 20SD (PCE Instruments, Meschede, Germany) was used to measure force during finger extension.

Flex Sensor: One 4.5 " Flex Sensor (Spectra Symbol, Salt Lake City, USA) was attached to the fingers with an adhesive strap.

Flex Sensor Reader: Flex sensors were connected to a microcontroller board (ATmega328P) over a voltage divider. Analog values from the flex sensor were sampled with 10 Hz and sent via USB to a PC.

Ortheses: Saebo Flex (Pro Walk, Egelsbach, Germany). To assess finger movement but not wrist extension patients were wearing an orthesis, stabilizing the wrist joint.

Stimulation Set-Up and Protocol

Four round electrodes were placed on top of the forearm extensor muscles. The indifferent electrode was placed close to the wrist. An orthesis stabilized the wrist joint. An adhesive strap was used to attach the index, middle and ring finger via a string and spring to the force gauge. Additionally, a flex sensor was attached to the hand with adhesive tape and allowed to slide under the adhesive strap. The arm was positioned in a slightly elevated position and fixated to avoid convulsions of the arm effecting the force measurement. Figure 7.1 illustrates the set-up used in this study.

Single pulses were applied to successively to determine which of the electrodes elicits the greatest finger extension. 6 blocks of stimulation (25 Hz and 25 mA) were applied with increasing pulse width (2 x 200, 2 x 250 and 2 x 300 µs). Pulse width was increased throughout the protocol to counter fatigue at least partly, allowing data collection also

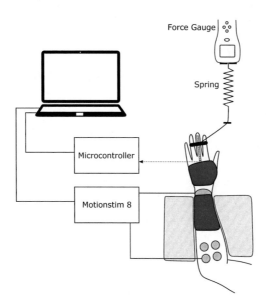

Fig. 7.1. Experimental set up for assessment of hand opening. The index, middle and ring finger are attached with a string and a spring to a force gauge. A flex sensor was attached to the ring finger.

for later blocks. Each block consisted of 10 stimulation phases with a duration of 10 s and 10 s pauses. Between each block was a three minute break.

Before and after the protocol the spasticity of the participant was assessed by a trained occupational therapist. Moreover, the force necessary to open the hand before and after the protocol was measured.

7.1.2 Results

As expected the stimulation induced force production and finger extension showed a significant reduction over time which correlates to our experiences of rapid occurring fatigue during repetitive electrical stimulation. The reduced effectiveness was already visible within the first three minutes of applied stimulation. However, spasticity of the flexor was lower after the stimulation protocol and less force was required to open the hand.

7.1.3 Conclusion

The very rapid decline in stimulation effect in individuals with chronic strokes observed in this study strongly underlines the necessity of methods to reduce neuromuscular fatigue during electrical stimulation. A manual adjustment of stimulation parameters to counter fatigue cannot be expected from patients or therapists without extensive training. Smart systems appear necessary to enable integration of electrical stimulation in functional neuroprosthesis.

A reduction of spasticity after electrical stimulation occurred which is a welcome side effect and was appreciated by the participants.

7.2 Effective Electrical Stimulation using Short Stimulation Pulses

Section 4.1 pointed out several advantages provided by electrical stimulation with short pulse widths. These considerations were based on theoretical calculations and simulations. Here, an assessment of short pulse efficiency shall be presented to judge whether short pulse width stimulation is suited for clinical applications. This study was performed in cooperation with the Department of Neurology of the University Medical Center Hamburg-Eppendorf.

7.2.1 Methods

In this study two different experiments were performed. Experiment 1 (efficiency comparison) assessed the stimulation effect of short (60 μs) and long (300 μs) pulse widths to determine whether short pulses show similar efficiency compared to longer pulses that are more frequently used. The stimulation effect on the extensor digitorum muscles was investigated for repetitive and continuous stimulation with 60 μs and 300 μs pulses.

Experiment 2 (comfort comparison) compared the discomfort caused during stimulation with 60, 180 and 300 μs pulses. Additionally, the peak voltage drop and electric charge that occurred during the stimulations were observed.

All stimulations were performed with a frequency of 25 Hz.

Subjects

10 healthy participants (mean age 30.7 years +/- 6.7 SD, 2 female) and 2 male individuals with chronic stroke took part in experiment 1 (efficiency comparison). 7 healthy participants (mean age 26.4 years +/- 2.1 SD, 1 female) participated in experiment 2 (comfort comparison). All participants gave written informed consent according to the Declaration of Helsinki. The study was approved by the local ethics committee of the Medical Association of Hamburg (PV4618).

Material

Stimulation Device: The MOTIONSTIM 8 (Section 5.4.1) was used in both experiments and stimulations were triggered using its digital inputs.

Stimulation Electrodes: Pals (Axelgaard, Fallbrook, CA, USA) electrodes were used in both experiments. The indifferent electrode was elliptic 4 x 6 cm^2, the active electrode (experiment 2) round with a 3.2 cm diameter.

Electrode Array: One array electrode (Section 4.4.1) was used for experiment 1.

Demultiplexer: Switchbox 1 (Section 5.2.1) was used to distribute the stimulation current to the electrode array.

Flex Sensor: One 4.5 " flex sensor (Spectra Symbol, Salt Lake City, USA) was attached to the observed finger with custom made rings.

Flex Sensor Reader and Stimulator Control: Flex sensors were connected to a microcontroller board (ATmega328P) over a voltage divider. Analog values from the flex sensor were sampled with 100 Hz. The median of the analog values was calculated for 10 samples and send via USB to a PC, thus resulting in a 10 Hz data stream. The microcontroller was additionally used to start and stop the stimulation blocks.

Stimulation Set-Up and Protocol

Efficiency Comparison An array electrode was placed on top of the forearm extensor muscles. The indifferent electrode was placed close to the wrist. An electrode search protocol was performed and the stimulation effect was evaluated visually to find the most effective electrode on the array. Seven single electrodes of the array were activated subsequently for 3 seconds with a 3 second pause in between. After the search protocol a flex sensor was attached either to the index, middle or ring finger, depending on which one showed the strongest extension. The stimulation amplitude necessary to achieve a finger extension that was easy to detect and caused as little discomfort as possible was determined for 60 and 300 μs pulses. Figure 7.2 illustrates the set-up used in the efficiency comparison.

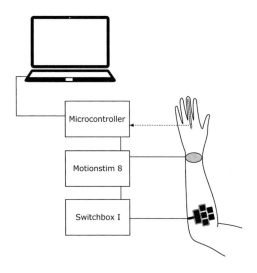

Fig. 7.2. Experimental set up for pulse width comparison.

The stimulation protocol was divided in two trials, each containing four stimulation blocks with a length of 130 s each. Two kinds of stimulation blocks were performed: first, continuous stimulation for 110 s, with 10 s breaks at the beginning and the end (cont.), second, repetitive stimulation with alternating phases of 8 s stimulation and 4 s rest (10 times) and a 10 s rest at the beginning (rep.). Each kind of block was either performed with a pulse width of 60 μs or 300 μs.

The order of blocks was: cont. 300, cont. 60, rep. 60, rep. 300, cont. 60, cont. 300, rep. 300, rep. 60. The participants had a two minute break between each block.

It was tried to start all blocks with a comparable finger extension, thus stimulation intensity was increased quickly at the beginning of a block if the achieved range of motion was too small.

Comfort Comparison   A round active electrode was placed over the finger extensor muscles to produce a extension of the index, middle or ring finger. The indifferent electrode was placed close to the wrist. A flex sensor was attached to the finger showing the greatest range of motion during initial tests.

Three different pulse widths were examined: 60, 180 and 300 μs. The amplitude was adjusted to produce the same level of extension for all pulse widths that were used. Nine blocks of 15 s stimulations were applied to the participant in a random manner (three of each pulse width).

Data Analysis

Efficiency Comparison - Healthy   Data evaluation was performed with a custom written Matlab program. The mean sensor value of the 10 s rest before the start of the stimulation was subtracted from all sensor values. The sensor values were normalized for each block by the maximum sensor value. Sensor values from continuous stimulation blocks were averaged into 11 phases of 10 s stimulation. Sensor values from repetitive stimulation blocks were averaged for each stimulation phase (10 hand openings). To asses statistical significant differences between 60 and 300 µs stimulation the mean hand opening over each 10 s phase (continuous stimulation), respectively single hand opening (repetitive stimulation), was determined. A paired two-sample t-test was used to evaluate the null hypothesis that the two data vectors are from populations with equal means, without assuming equal variance of the two populations.

Efficiency Comparison - Stroke   An individual evaluation of data from individuals with stroke was performed. The fatigue time was compared for continuous stimulation and the number of full contractions for repetitive stimulation. The time it took for a sensor value to drop below 70.7 % of the maximum sensor value during that block was defined as the fatigue time [110]. Movements, producing sensor values above 70.7 % of the first hand opening in the stimulation block, were defined as full contractions.

Comfort Comparison   Participants were asked to grade the comfort of the stimulation on a visual analog scale (VAS) without seeing the previous answers after each stimulation block. A range from pleasant (0) to painful (10) was used for the VAS. An oscilloscope monitored the peak voltage drop during the 15 s stimulation. For each participant median comfort level and mean peak voltage were determined. A paired two-sample t-test was used to evaluate the alternative hypothesis that the population mean of discomfort for 60 µs is less than for 180, or 300 µs.

7.2.2 Results

Efficiency Comparison - Healthy The two-sample t-test rejected the null hypothesis that the population mean for 60 μs and 300 μs pulses are equal for trial 2 of continuous stimulation (p < 0.01) and trial 1 (p < 0.01) and trial 2 (p < 0.01) of repetitive stimulation (Figure 7.3). The null hypothesis was not rejected for trial 1 of continuous stimulation (p > 0.05).

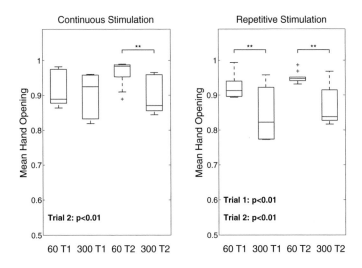

Fig. 7.3. Box plots of mean sensor values. The mean was calculated over all subjects. Box plots show distribution of values over time. Asterisks mark significance level with (*) p<0.05 and (**) p<0.01.

The size of the boxes in Figure 7.3 represents the spread of sensor values during stimulation blocks. The observed spread of sensor values was smaller for stimulation with 60 μs pulse width compared to 300 μs pulse width, especially for repetitive stimulation.

Figure 7.4 and 7.5 show boxplots illustrating the variation of hand opening among subjects for continuous and repetitive stimulation.

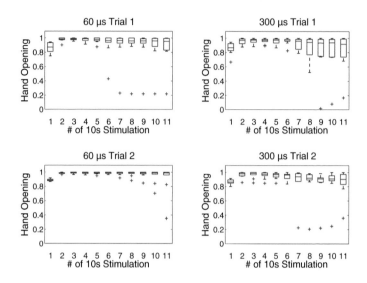

Fig. 7.4. Box plots of continuous stimulation with 60 and 300 μs pulses. Sensor values were normalized for each subject. Mean data of 11 10s periods is compared.

Efficiency Comparison - Stroke   Evaluating the data from individuals with stroke did not show a significant difference between 60 and 300 μs pulse widths (Table 7.1). Patient 1 did not show different fatigue times for continuous stimulation with 60 or 300 μs pulses, since finger extension remained constant throughout the measurements. Patient 2 showed an early onset of fatigue (38.4 s) already in the first block of continuous stimulation (60 μs). In the second block of continuous stimulation (300 μs) the fatigue time was even lower (28.0 s). During trial 2 no evaluable data could be generated, since discomfort with 300 μs pulses did not allow to increase the stimulation intensity to offset the reduced stimulation effect probably caused by neuromuscular fatigue.

Repetitive stimulation data showed mixed results, with Patient 1 having a slightly better performance with 300 μs pulses, whereas Patient 2 had a better outcome with 60 μs pulses.

Comfort Comparison   Participants reported significant less discomfort during 60 μs pulse width stimulation compared to 180 and 300 μs (Figure 7.6 (a)). Using longer pulse

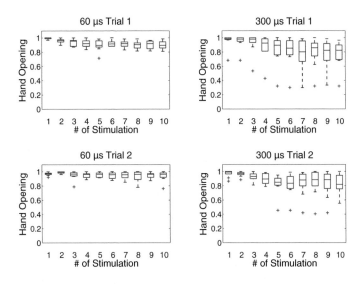

Fig. 7.5. Box plots of repetitive stimulation with 60 and 300 µs pulses. Sensor values were normalized for each subject. Mean data for each stimulation block is compared.

Tab. 7.1. Fatigue time and number of contractions and for individuals with stroke. '-' indicates that sensor data could not be evaluated. 'max' means a complete finger extension was observed for the entire 110 s of stimulation.

	Pulse Width	Patient 1	Patient 2
Fatigue Time	60 µs	max / max	28.0 s / -
	300 µs	max / max	38.4 s / -
# Contractions	60 µs	5 / 10	8 / 4
	300 µs	10 / 10	2 / -

widths resulted in a decreased necessary amplitude ($I_{60} = 20.67\,\text{mA}$, $I_{180} = 13.71\,\text{mA}$, $I_{300} = 11.86\,\text{mA}$), however, peak voltage ($V_{60} = 50.3\,\text{V}$, $V_{180} = 57.7\,\text{V}$, $V_{300} = 60.2\,\text{V}$) and charge ($Q_{60} = 1.24\,\mu\text{C}$, $Q_{180} = 2.47\,\mu\text{C}$, $Q_{300} = 3.56\,\mu\text{C}$) increased (Figure 7.6 (b)).

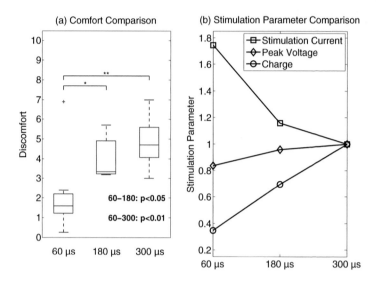

Fig. 7.6. Boxplot of discomfort and peak voltage for different pulse widths (a). Asterisks mark significance level with (*) $p<0.05$ and (**) $p<0.01$. Comparison of the mean stimulation parameters, normalized at $300\,\mu\text{s}$ (b).

7.2.3 Discussion

A decreasing stimulation effect was observed for 60 and $300\,\mu\text{s}$ pulses in continuous and repetitive stimulation. It could already be shown that electrical stimulation with short pulse width is an effective method in charge reduction. It was now investigated whether short charge efficient pulses are able to achieve the same stimulation effect compared to more classical pulse widths. Measurements with healthy subjects demonstrated a weaker decrease of stimulation effect for $60\,\mu\text{s}$ pulses compared to $300\,\mu\text{s}$ pulses. Data from individuals with chronic stroke, however, did not provide evidence that one pulse width performs superior compared to the other. Albeit, one stroke survivor showed little tolerance for long pulse width stimulation, limiting the range of motion that could be achieved.

A comfort comparison performed with 7 healthy subjects showed a significantly reduced discomfort with short pulse width stimulation. Only one subject, who had no previous contact with electrical stimulation, reported more discomfort with short stimulation pulses.

Naturally, electrical stimulation with short pulse widths requires higher amplitudes, nevertheless, the peak voltage drop during short stimulation pulses was lower.

7.3 Smart Intensity Control with DLFS - a Demonstration

In Section 6.3.1 a sensor based intensity control was presented. The idea behind this approach was to enable an algorithm to counter the rapid onset of neuromuscular fatigue during electrical stimulation. Distributed low frequency stimulation (DLFS, Section 4.3.3) is one technique reported to delay the onset of stimulation induced fatigue. Here, the effect of smart intensity control will be demonstrated, moreover, DLFS is added in some measurements to see whether the performance can be increased with this technique.

7.3.1 Methods

In this demonstration continuous and repetitive stimulation was used to show the efficacy of the smart intensity control. Stimulation was applied in six blocks, four blocks using continuous stimulation and two blocks with repetitive stimulation. In two continuous stimulation blocks DLFS was performed to assess whether the onset of neuromuscular fatigue can be delayed this way. It was examined whether the smart intensity control is able to maintain a continuous stable hand opening and whether repeated hand openings with the same range of motion can be achieved.

Subjects

9 healthy participants (mean age 29.33 years +/- 12.72 SD, 4 female) took part in this study. All participants gave written informed consent according to the Declaration of Helsinki. The study was approved by the local ethics committee of the Medical Association of Hamburg (PV4618).

Material

Stimulation Device: The MOTIONSTIM 8 (Section 5.4.1) was used for this demonstration and stimulations were triggered using its digital inputs.

Stimulation Electrodes: A Pals 4 x 6 cm^2 elliptic (Axelgaard, Fallbrook, CA, USA) electrode was used as the indifferent electrode.

Electrode Array: Two array electrodes (Section 4.4.1) were used to find the optimal active electrodes.

Demultiplexer: Switchbox 1 (Section 5.2.1) was used to distribute the stimulation current to the electrode array and to allow DLFS. Additionally, results of the search protocols were send to a PC via USB.

Flex Sensor: Two 4.5 " flex sensors (Spectra Symbol, Salt Lake City, USA) were attached to the index and ring finger with custom made rings.

Flex Sensor Reader and Stimulator Control: Flex sensors were connected to a microcontroller board (ATmega328P) over a voltage divider. Analog values from the flex sensor were sampled with 100 Hz. The median of the analog values was calculated for 10 samples and sent via USB to a PC, thus resulting in a 10 Hz data stream. Additionally, the microcontroller was used for the smart intensity control.

Stimulation Set-Up and Protocol

Two array electrodes were placed on top of the forearm covering most of the extensor muscles. Two array electrodes were used this time to have a larger selection of possible stimulation sites, increasing the likelihood of finding two electrodes that produce a similar hand opening for DLFS. The indifferent electrode was placed close to the wrist. Two flex sensors were attached to hand, one to the index finger and another to the ring finger. A search protocol was performed and the sensor values were evaluated on a PC. Two electrodes eliciting a clear and comparable hand opening were then noted and used for DLFS. The better one of the two electrodes was used for normal single electrode stimulation. Figure 7.7 illustrates the set-up used for the demonstration.

The stimulation protocol was divided in two trials, each containing three blocks. Three kinds of stimulation blocks were performed: first, normal continuous stimulation for 110 s with one electrode (cont. norm.), second, continuous DLFS (cont. DLFS) and third, six repetitive stimulation with a duration of 10 s and 10 s pauses (rep.).
The order of blocks was: cont. norm., cont. DLFS, rep., cont. DLFS, cont. norm, rep..
The participants had a two minute break between each block.

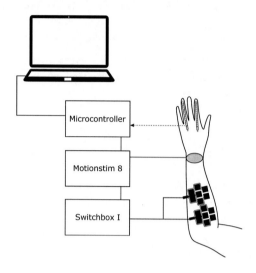

Fig. 7.7. Experimental set up for smart intensity control with distributed low frequency stimulation.

7.3.2 Results

Sensor data obtained from continuous stimulation was averaged into 10 s phases. Sensor values from repetitive stimulation blocks were averaged for each stimulation phase (6 hand openings). The smart intensity control enabled a complete hand opening well above 80 % for all participants during continuous stimulation (Figure 7.8 and Figure 7.9). This was true for normal stimulation with one electrode as well as DLFS. The mean pulse width increased for the second trials (Table 7.2). Additionally, DLFS required a slightly higher pulse width and more intensity increases (corrections) were required to maintain the hand open (Table 7.2). At least two corrections in one subject during DLFS were caused by a stimulation induced tremor (Figure 7.10).

During repetitive stimulation stable and repeatable hand openings could be achieved, even though some outliers were observed. (Figure 7.11). The outliers showed sensor values smaller than 80 % of the maximum extension in the respective block. The pulse width used during the smart intensity control showed a larger variation compared to the sensor values (Figure 7.12). In trial 2 an increase in required pulse width can be observed for hand opening four to six.

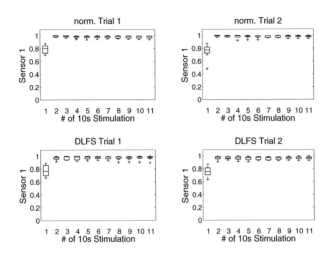

Fig. 7.8. Boxplots of values from sensor 1 during continuous stimulation with normal and distributed low frequency stimulation (DLFS).

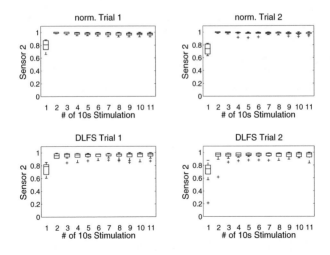

Fig. 7.9. Boxplots of values from sensor 2 during continuous stimulation with normal and distributed low frequency stimulation (DLFS).

Tab. 7.2. Pulse width and number of corrections during continuous stimulation with normal and distributed low frequency stimulation (DLFS).

	Normal Stimulation	DLFS
Mean Pulse Width [µs]	72.8 / 77.1	73.3 / 77.4
# Corrections	1 / 2 (2 subjects)	3 (2 subjects) / 4 (3 subjects)

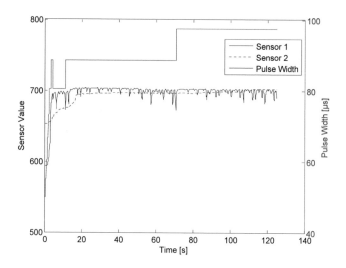

Fig. 7.10. Flex sensor values and stimulation pulse width during distributed low frequency stimulation with closed-loop intensity control. A stimulation induced finger tremor interferes with the intensity control and causes unnecessary increases in stimulation intensity.

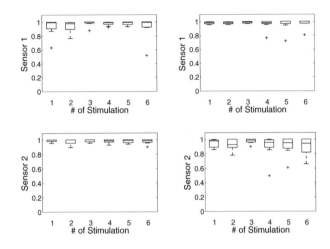

Fig. 7.11. Boxplots of sensor values during repetitive stimulation with smart intensity control.

7.3.3 Discussion

This demonstration showed that the smart intensity control described in Section 6.3.1 enables reliable continuous hand openings by detecting reductions of finger extensions and increasing the intensity accordingly.

Repetitive stimulation showed an overall stable performance but some outliers were observed. The smart intensity control used works without any previous calibration and determines an effective stimulation intensity and range of motion for each stimulation phase. Adding more strict minimum extensions and adjusting the threshold values for effective stimulation could prevent the outliers present in this demonstration. Another possibility is using a calibration based intensity control (Section 6.3.2) which would probably lead to even more robust results. Whether DLFS is a practical way to increase the effect of FES of the hand remains to be seen.

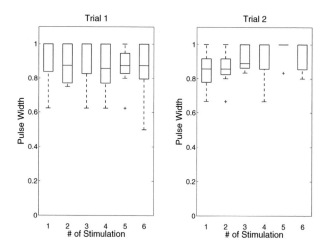

Fig. 7.12. Boxplots of pulse width during repetitive stimulation with smart intensity control.

7.4 General Considerations Regarding Application of FES

As a preparation for the studies presented in this chapter preliminary experiments were performed. In this section general considerations and feedback of patients that were gathered during preliminary experiments and the performed studies shall be discussed.

7.4.1 Electrode Placement

The correct placement of electrodes, especially for patients at home or personnel without a medical background is a challenging task. The use of a pen electrode proved to be extremely valuable during preliminary experiments. Also the use of an external switch to start and stop stimulation phases at will eases the process of determining effective sites for electrode placement compared to cyclic stimulation programs.

Something else to consider is the electrode geometry which has shown a non-negligible effect on stimulation efficacy and was therefore examined by simulations and experiments (section 4.2). In later studies electrode arrays were used, which eased the whole process of determining sites for electrode placement tremendously. However, usability for elder people at home is something that has to be optimized to allow this technology to have a real long term impact on the way FES is going to be applied in the future.

7.4.2 Patient Training Participation

FES as a mean to facilitate recovery after a stroke benefits greatly from active training participation. Elicited movements and the patients' intention have to happen synchronously to support restructuring mechanisms in the motor cortex. In a preliminary experiment with a stroke survivor active participation was tried to be achieved with a direct intensity control using a gaming joystick. The subject could perform two different movements with the joystick, hand and finger extension as well as flexion, while being able to adjust the grade of stimulation intensity. It could be observed that the subject was able to handle the joystick but was not using the option to regulate the stimulation intensity; stimulation intensity was always chosen to be at zero or at the maximum possible intensity. Also stimulation of the finger flexors was of little interest for the subject, most likely due to the fact that the subjects forearm extensor muscles were paralyzed the most, which is very common for stroke survivors. This preliminary test as well as interviews with stroke survivors and therapists during the course of the whole project led to the conclusion that even though active participation is very important, it has to be achieved in an intuitive and easy manner, e.g. through techniques similar to the ones described in section 6.2.

7.5 Experimental Findings - Conclusion

In the studies presented here a decreasing effect of electrical stimulation over time was found, underlining the importance of techniques to counter this effect, especially for neuroprosthesis used on a daily basis. Short pulse width stimulation demonstrated a gentle method to perform FES of the hand, potentially even reducing neuromuscular fatigue. Together with feedback based intensity control reliable and robust movements could be generated, hopefully improving the application of FES in the future.

8 Conclusion

This thesis covers a broad spectrum of topics related to the field of electrical stimulation of neural tissue by surface electrodes. The focus lay on systems improving the daily life of individuals suffering from impaired hand functions caused by stroke. The success of electrical stimulation is often limited by difficulties during the placement of electrodes, an early onset of neuromuscular fatigue and no available methods for an intuitive and automated control of the stimulation process. These limitations were always kept in mind during the scope of this thesis.

To gain a deep understanding of fundamental mechanisms underlying the process of electrical stimulation and its effect on biological tissue a simulation environment was designed from the ground up. The simulation environment, in form of a two-step approach containing a 3D FE model on the one hand and mathematical representations of motor axons on the other, allowed the prediction of neural reactions to stimuli applied by surface electrodes. The versatility of this simulation method enabled the investigation of topics related to the efficiency of electrical stimulation, directly influencing following developments. The validity of the presented simulation environment is, of course, limited by the fact that lumped and FE models only represent a simplified version of real physiological behavior. Therefore, simulation results can only be the first step for the design of new treatment paradigms.

Studying the efficiency of stimulation pulses revealed several benefits of short stimulation pulses. Later, an experimental study supported these findings and indicated that short pulse width stimulation can be used for charge efficient, comfortable and selective electrical stimulation of the hand, potentially also reducing neuromuscular fatigue.

The influence of electrode geometry on force generation could be understood thanks to simulations and the found importance of axon orientation was considered in the design of electrode arrays by the use of square or round electrodes. The effect of electrode to electrode distance and hydrogel resistivity are things that can be assessed with stimulations as well.

A novel method to fabricate electrode arrays was developed during this project for rapid prototyping. Using a commercial ink-jet printer to print patterns of conductive silver on a polymer substrate allows a fast and cheap production of electrode arrays with customizable electrode number, distribution and geometry.

Hardware to demultiplex the stimulation current is needed to perform electrical stimulation with electrode arrays. Two systems to perform electrical stimulation with electrode arrays were presented. At first a simple system that can be used with any stimulation device was developed. Later a distinct improvement of this system was introduced that enables multi-channel stimulation together with a wireless control over a smartphone or tablet. The interface of the stimulation system was developed in a way to allow an easy and safe control of electrical stimulation with electrode arrays, thereby tremendously simplifying the process to determine effective stimulation sites.

Sensors or biosignals offer the possibility to trigger stimulation events in an intuitive way to enable real-life applications and natural training protocols to relearn lost functions. These can be as simple as opening the hand to hold a wallet. Still, such functions can have a great impact on the quality of life for impaired patients. It was demonstrated how finger extension and EMG signals, acquired by external systems connected wirelessly to the smartphone, can be used to start and stop stimulation events. Sensor data can also be used to provide feedback of the stimulation induced movements. This information was used in two examples to build feedback based controls of the stimulation intensity. An intelligent and automated intensity control offers a great assistance to the patient and can also be utilized to offset the decreasing effect of electrical stimulation over time, by adjusting the stimulation intensity accordingly. Feedback controlled stimulation in conjunction with means of control adjusted to the impairment of the patient offer the foundation for future neuroprosthesis.

Outlook

To finalize the systems presented in this thesis, clinical studies involving impaired patients are necessary to ensure high acceptance and quality of life improvements.

A new stimulation device, specifically designed for the integration in a smartphone controlled neuroprosthesis, could be developed. This device could be miniaturized to a certain extent by sacrificing the display and control elements. The functions of the

Smartstim adapter should be included directly into the device. More important than miniaturizing the stimulation hardware are the software as well as the communication protocol. A risk analysis has to be performed to identify possible security flaws and to ensure a safe operation under every condition.

An industrialized process to manufacture electrode arrays is necessary for a final product. An industrial fabrication process could involve screen printed electrodes using medical silver/silver chloride paste and an insulating coating.

The final system requires an orthesis which is easy to apply and contains the electrode array. The demultiplexer and a sensor system could also be included in such an orthesis, while the miniaturized stimulator could be worn on the upper arm.

Even though no commercial product can be generated immediately the here presented systems can be used conveniently for further research activities.

To offer stimulation results exceeding the possibilities of electrode arrays implanted electrode systems are a possible field of research in the future.

List of Figures

List of Tables

References

[1] S.-M. Lai, S. Studenski, P. W. Duncan, and S. Perera, "Persisting consequences of stroke measured by the stroke impact scale", *Stroke*, vol. 33, no. 7, pp. 1840–1844, 2002. DOI: 10.1161/01.str.0000019289.15440.f2 (cit. on p. 1).

[2] L. A. Benton, L. L. Baker, B. R. Bowman, and R. L. Waters, *Funktionelle Elektrostimulation: Ein Leitfaden für die Praxis (German Edition)*. Steinkopff, 1983, ISBN: 3-7985-0622-1 (cit. on pp. 1, 11).

[3] F. Quandt and F. C. Hummel, "The influence of functional electrical stimulation on hand motor recovery in stroke patients: A review", *Experimental & Translational Stroke Medicine*, vol. 6, no. 1, p. 9, 2014. DOI: 10.1186/2040-7378-6-9 (cit. on pp. 1, 85).

[4] L. L. Baker, C. Yeh, D. Wilson, and R. L. Waters, "Electrical stimulation of wrist and fingers for hemiplegic patients.", *Physical therapy*, vol. 59, pp. 1495–1499, 12 Dec. 1979, ISSN: 0031-9023 (cit. on p. 1).

[5] B. M. Doucet, A. Lam, L. Griffin, *et al.*, "Neuromuscular electrical stimulation for skeletal muscle function", *Yale J Biol Med*, vol. 85, no. 2, 2012 (cit. on pp. 1, 11, 85, 86).

[6] M. Popovic, T. Keller, I. Papas, V. Dietz, and M. Morari, "Surface-stimulation technology for grasping and walking neuroprostheses", *IEEE Engineering in Medicine and Biology Magazine*, vol. 20, no. 1, pp. 82–93, 2001. DOI: 10.1109/51.897831 (cit. on pp. 1, 86, 89).

[7] N. M. Malešević, L. Z. Maneski, V. Ilić, N. Jorgovanović, G. Bijelić, T. Keller, and D. B. Popović, "A multi-pad electrode based functional electrical stimulation system for restoration of grasp", *Journal of NeuroEngineering and Rehabilitation*, vol. 9, no. 1, p. 66, 2012. DOI: 10.1186/1743-0003-9-66 (cit. on pp. 1, 53, 58, 81–83).

[8]   R. Rupp, A. Kreilinger, M. Rohm, V. Kaiser, and G. R. Muller-Putz, "Develop-
      ment of a non-invasive, multifunctional grasp neuroprosthesis and its evaluation
      in an individual with a high spinal cord injury", in *2012 Annual International
      Conference of the IEEE Engineering in Medicine and Biology Society*, Institute
      of Electrical and Electronics Engineers (IEEE), 2012. DOI: 10.1109/embc.
      2012.6346308 (cit. on pp. 1, 86).

[9]   M. Štrbac, S. Kočović, M. Marković, and D. B. Popović, "Microsoft kinect-
      based artificial perception system for control of functional electrical stimulation
      assisted grasping", *BioMed Research International*, vol. 2014, pp. 1–12, 2014.
      DOI: 10.1155/2014/740469 (cit. on p. 1).

[10] D. B. Popović and M. B. Popović, "Automatic determination of the optimal
      shape of a surface electrode: Selective stimulation.", *Journal of neuroscience
      methods*, vol. 178, pp. 174–181, 1 Mar. 2009, ISSN: 0165-0270. DOI: 10.1016/j.
      jneumeth.2008.12.003 (cit. on pp. 1, 53, 54).

[11] M. Rohm, M. Schneiders, C. Müller, A. Kreilinger, V. Kaiser, G. R. Müller-Putz,
      and R. Rupp, "Hybrid brain–computer interfaces and hybrid neuroprostheses
      for restoration of upper limb functions in individuals with high-level spinal cord
      injury", *Artificial Intelligence in Medicine*, vol. 59, no. 2, pp. 133–142, 2013.
      DOI: 10.1016/j.artmed.2013.07.004 (cit. on pp. 1, 87).

[12] B. Smith, P. H. Peckham, M. W. Keith, and D. D. Roscoe, "An externally
      powered, multichannel, implantable stimulator for versatile control of paralyzed
      muscle", *IEEE Transactions on Biomedical Engineering*, vol. BME-34, no. 7,
      pp. 499–508, 1987. DOI: 10.1109/tbme.1987.325979 (cit. on pp. 1, 86).

[13] J. S. Knutson, M. Y. Harley, T. Z. Hisel, and J. Chae, "Improving hand function
      in stroke survivors: A pilot study of contralaterally controlled functional electric
      stimulation in chronic hemiplegia", *Archives of Physical Medicine and Rehabil-
      itation*, vol. 88, no. 4, pp. 513–520, 2007. DOI: 10.1016/j.apmr.2007.01.003
      (cit. on pp. 1, 85).

[14] J. S. Knutson, M. Y. Harley, T. Z. Hisel, N. S. Makowski, M. J. Fu, and J. Chae,
      "Contralaterally controlled functional electrical stimulation for stroke rehabili-
      tation", in *2012 Annual International Conference of the IEEE Engineering in
      Medicine and Biology Society*, Institute of Electrical and Electronics Engineers
      (IEEE), 2012. DOI: 10.1109/embc.2012.6345932 (cit. on pp. 1, 85).

[15] D. C. Irimia, M. S. Poboroniuc, S. Hartopanu, D. Sticea, G. Paicu, and B. E. Ignat, "Post-stroke hand rehabilitation using a hybrid FES-robotic glove", in *2016 International Conference and Exposition on Electrical and Power Engineering (EPE)*, Institute of Electrical and Electronics Engineers (IEEE), 2016. DOI: 10.1109/icepe.2016.7781362 (cit. on p. 1).

[16] H. Kim, G. Lee, and C. Song, "Effect of functional electrical stimulation with mirror therapy on upper extremity motor function in poststroke patients", *Journal of Stroke and Cerebrovascular Diseases*, vol. 23, no. 4, pp. 655–661, 2014. DOI: 10.1016/j.jstrokecerebrovasdis.2013.06.017 (cit. on pp. 1, 85).

[17] M. Santos, L. H. Zahner, B. J. McKiernan, J. D. Mahnken, and B. Quaney, "Neuromuscular electrical stimulation improves severe hand dysfunction for individuals with chronic stroke", *Journal of Neurologic Physical Therapy*, vol. 30, no. 4, pp. 175–183, 2006. DOI: 10.1097/01.npt.0000281254.33045.e4 (cit. on p. 1).

[18] J. Eraifej, W. Clark, B. France, S. Desando, and D. Moore, "Effectiveness of upper limb functional electrical stimulation after stroke for the improvement of activities of daily living and motor function: A systematic review and meta-analysis", *Systematic Reviews*, vol. 6, no. 1, 2017. DOI: 10.1186/s13643-017-0435-5 (cit. on p. 1).

[19] Bioness, *NESS H200*, URL: https://www.bioness.com/Products/H200_for_Hand_Paralysis.php, Accessed: 13 April 2018 (cit. on p. 2).

[20] A. Popović-Bijelić, G. Bijelić, N. Jorgovanović, D. Bojanić, M. B. Popović, and D. B. Popović, "Multi-field surface electrode for selective electrical stimulation.", *Artificial organs*, vol. 29, pp. 448–452, 6 Jun. 2005, ISSN: 0160-564X. DOI: 10.1111/j.1525-1594.2005.29075.x (cit. on p. 2).

[21] T. Keller and A. Kuhn, "Electrodes for transcutaneous (surface) electrical stimulation", *Journal of Automatic Control*, vol. 18, no. 2, pp. 35–45, 2008. DOI: 10.2298/jac0802035k (cit. on pp. 2, 22, 53, 58).

[22] M. Boulos, S. Wheeler, C. Tavares, and R. Jones, "How smartphones are changing the face of mobile and participatory healthcare: An overview, with example from eCAALYX", *BioMedical Engineering OnLine*, vol. 10, no. 1, p. 24, 2011. DOI: 10.1186/1475-925x-10-24 (cit. on p. 2).

[23] A. W. G. Buijink, B. J. Visser, and L. Marshall, "Medical apps for smartphones: Lack of evidence undermines quality and safety", *Evidence Based Medicine*, vol. 18, no. 3, pp. 90–92, 2012. DOI: 10.1136/eb-2012-100885 (cit. on p. 2).

[24] A. Faller and M. Schünke, *Der Körper des Menschen: Einführung in Bau und Funktion*. Thieme, 2008, ISBN: 978-3-13-329715-8 (cit. on p. 3).

[25] G. Thews, E. Mutschler, and P. Vaupel, *Anatomie, Physiologie, Pathophysiologie des Menschen*. Wissenschaftliche Verlagsges., 1999, ISBN: 3-8047-1616-4 (cit. on p. 3).

[26] K. Golenhofen, *Basislehrbuch Physiologie*. Urban + Fischer, 2004, ISBN: 3-437-42481-5 (cit. on pp. 3, 4).

[27] P. Husar, *Biosignalverarbeitung*. Springer Berlin Heidelberg, Jul. 23, 2010. [Online]. Available: http://www.ebook.de/de/product/19110827/peter_husar_biosignalverarbeitung.html (cit. on p. 3).

[28] M. Frotscher and W. Kahle, *Color Atlas of Human Anatomy: Nervous System and Sensory Organs*. Thieme, 2010, ISBN: 978-3-13-533506-3 (cit. on p. 3).

[29] L. A. Saleh, *Implant System for the Recording of Internal Muscle Activity to Control a Hand Prosthesis (Wissenschaftliche Beitrage Zur Medizinelektronik)*. Logos Verlag Berlin, 2015, ISBN: 978-3-8325-4153-8 (cit. on p. 10).

[30] M. Gobbo, N. A. Maffiuletti, C. Orizio, and M. A. Minetto, "Muscle motor point identification is essential for optimizing neuromuscular electrical stimulation use", *Journal of NeuroEngineering and Rehabilitation*, vol. 11, no. 1, p. 17, 2014. DOI: 10.1186/1743-0003-11-17 (cit. on p. 16).

[31] A. L. Hodgkin and A. F. Huxley, "A quantitative description of membrane current and its application to conduction and excitation in nerve", *The Journal of Physiology*, vol. 117, no. 4, pp. 500–544, 1952. DOI: 10.1113/jphysiol.1952.sp004764 (cit. on pp. 17, 24, 29).

[32] A. Kuhn, "Modeling transcutaneous electrical stimulation", PhD thesis, ETH ZURICH, 2008 (cit. on pp. 17, 27, 50).

[33] *COMSOL Multiphysics User's Guide*, COMSOL 4.3, May 2012 (cit. on p. 18).

[34] *AC/DC Module User's Guide*, COMSOL 4.3b, May 2013 (cit. on p. 18).

[35] D. L. Villarreal, D. Schroeder, and W. H. Krautschneider, "Equivalent circuit model to simulate the neuromuscular electrical stimulation", in *ICT.Open*, 2013 (cit. on p. 18).

[36] S. Joucla and B. Yvert, "Modeling extracellular electrical neural stimulation: From basic understanding to MEA-based applications", *Journal of Physiology-Paris*, vol. 106, no. 3-4, pp. 146–158, 2012. DOI: 10.1016/j.jphysparis.2011.10.003 (cit. on p. 21).

[37] C. A. Bossetti, M. J. Birdno, and W. M. Grill, "Analysis of the quasi-static approximation for calculating potentials generated by neural stimulation", *Journal of Neural Engineering*, vol. 5, no. 1, pp. 44–53, 2007. DOI: 10.1088/1741-2560/5/1/005 (cit. on p. 21).

[38] A. Kuhn, T. Keller, M. Lawrence, and M. Morari, "A model for transcutaneous current stimulation: Simulations and experiments", *Medical & Biological Engineering & Computing*, vol. 47, no. 3, pp. 279–289, 2008. DOI: 10.1007/s11517-008-0422-z (cit. on pp. 21, 22).

[39] K. R. Foster and H. P. Schwan, "Dielectric properties of tissues and biological materials: A critical review.", *Critical reviews in biomedical engineering*, vol. 17, pp. 25–104, 1 1989, ISSN: 0278-940X (cit. on p. 22).

[40] S Gabriel, R. W. Lau, and C Gabriel, "The dielectric properties of biological tissues: III. parametric models for the dielectric spectrum of tissues", *Physics in Medicine and Biology*, vol. 41, no. 11, pp. 2271–2293, 1996. DOI: 10.1088/0031-9155/41/11/003 (cit. on p. 22).

[41] C. Polk and E. Postow, *CRC Handbook of Biological Effects of Electromagnetic Fields*. CRC Press, 1986, ISBN: 0849332656 (cit. on p. 22).

[42] J. P. Reilly, *Applied Bioelectricity*. Springer Nature, 1998. DOI: 10.1007/978-1-4612-1664-3 (cit. on p. 22).

[43] D. R. McNeal, "Analysis of a model for excitation of myelinated nerve", *IEEE Transactions on Biomedical Engineering*, vol. BME-23, no. 4, pp. 329–337, 1976. DOI: 10.1109/tbme.1976.324593 (cit. on pp. 24, 25, 27, 29–31).

[44] B. Frankenhaeuser and A. F. Huxley, "The action potential in the myelinated nerve fibre ofXenopus laevisas computed on the basis of voltage clamp data", *The Journal of Physiology*, vol. 171, no. 2, pp. 302–315, 1964. DOI: 10.1113/jphysiol.1964.sp007378 (cit. on pp. 24, 29–31).

[45] J. D. Gomez-Tames, J. Gonzalez, S. Nakamura, and W. Yu, "Simulation of the muscle recruitment by transcutaneous electrical stimulation in a simplified semitendinosus muscle model", in *Converging Clinical and Engineering Research*

on Neurorehabilitation, Springer Nature, 2013, pp. 449–453. DOI: 10.1007/978-3-642-34546-3_73 (cit. on pp. 27, 33, 36).

[46] F. Rattay, "Analysis of models for external stimulation of axons", *IEEE Transactions on Biomedical Engineering*, vol. BME-33, no. 10, pp. 974–977, 1986. DOI: 10.1109/tbme.1986.325670 (cit. on p. 25).

[47] F Rattay, "Modeling the excitation of fibers under surface electrodes.", *IEEE transactions on bio-medical engineering*, vol. 35, pp. 199–202, 3 Mar. 1988, ISSN: 0018-9294. DOI: 10.1109/10.1362 (cit. on p. 25).

[48] S. Y. Chiu, J. M. Ritchie, R. B. Rogart, and D Stagg, "A quantitative description of membrane currents in rabbit myelinated nerve.", *The Journal of Physiology*, vol. 292, no. 1, pp. 149–166, 1979. DOI: 10.1113/jphysiol.1979.sp012843 (cit. on p. 29).

[49] A. G. Richardson, C. C. McIntyre, and W. M. Grill, "Modelling the effects of electric fields on nerve fibres: Influence of the myelin sheath", *Medical & Biological Engineering & Computing*, vol. 38, no. 4, pp. 438–446, 2000. DOI: 10.1007/bf02345014 (cit. on p. 29).

[50] C. C. McIntyre, A. G. Richardson, and W. M. Grill, "Modeling the excitability of mammalian nerve fibers: Influence of afterpotentials on the recovery cycle", *Journal of neurophysiology*, vol. 87, no. 2, pp. 995–1006, 2002 (cit. on p. 29).

[51] K Saitou, T Masuda, D Michikami, R Kojima, and M Okada, "Innervation zones of the upper and lower limb muscles estimated by using multichannel surface emg.", *Journal of human ergology*, vol. 29, pp. 35–52, 1-2 Dec. 2000, ISSN: 0300-8134 (cit. on p. 33).

[52] S. Jezernik and M. Morari, "Energy-optimal electrical excitation of nerve fibers", *IEEE Transactions on Biomedical Engineering*, vol. 52, no. 4, pp. 740–743, 2005. DOI: 10.1109/tbme.2005.844050 (cit. on p. 41).

[53] S. Jezernik, T. Sinkjaer, and M. Morari, "Charge and energy minimization in electrical/magnetic stimulation of nervous tissue", *Journal of Neural Engineering*, vol. 7, no. 4, p. 046004, 2010. DOI: 10.1088/1741-2560/7/4/046004 (cit. on p. 41).

[54] M. A. Meza-Cuevas, D. Schroeder, and W. H. Krautschneider, "Neuromuscular electrical stimulation using different waveforms: Properties comparison by applying single pulses", in *2012 5th International Conference on BioMedical*

Engineering and Informatics, Institute of Electrical and Electronics Engineers (IEEE), 2012. DOI: 10.1109/bmei.2012.6512988 (cit. on p. 41).

[55] N. I. Krouchev, S. M. Danner, A. Vinet, F. Rattay, and M. Sawan, "Energy-optimal electrical-stimulation pulses shaped by the least-action principle", *PLoS ONE*, vol. 9, no. 3, D. R. Chialvo, Ed., e90480, 2014. DOI: 10.1371/journal.pone.0090480 (cit. on pp. 41, 44).

[56] A. Reinert, J. C. Loitz, N. Remer, D. Schroeder, and W. H. Krautschnei-der, "Usability of passive models for energy minimization of transcutaneous electrical stimulation - possibilities and shortcomings of analytical solutions of passive models and possible improvements", in *Proceedings of the 9th International Joint Conference on Biomedical Engineering Systems and Technologies*, Scitepress, 2016. DOI: 10.5220/0005822402690274 (cit. on p. 41).

[57] J. C. Loitz, A. Reinert, N. Remer, D. Schroeder, and W. H. Krautschneider, "Energy minimization during transcutaneous electrical stimulation by charge efficient stimulation pulses - benefits of using short duration and high amplitude stimulation pulses", in *Proceedings of the 9th International Joint Conference on Biomedical Engineering Systems and Technologies*, Scitepress, 2016. DOI: 10.5220/0005814202510255 (cit. on p. 42).

[58] D. R. Merrill, M. Bikson, and J. G. Jefferys, "Electrical stimulation of excitable tissue: Design of efficacious and safe protocols", *Journal of Neuroscience Methods*, vol. 141, no. 2, pp. 171–198, 2005. DOI: 10.1016/j.jneumeth.2004.10.020 (cit. on pp. 43, 44).

[59] W. Grill and J. Mortimer, "The effect of stimulus pulse duration on selectivity of neural stimulation", *IEEE Transactions on Biomedical Engineering*, vol. 43, no. 2, pp. 161–166, 1996. DOI: 10.1109/10.481985 (cit. on p. 45).

[60] J. C. Loitz, A. Reinert, D. Schroeder, and W. H. Krautschneider, "Impact of electrode geometry on force generation during functional electrical stimulation", *Current Directions in Biomedical Engineering*, vol. 1, no. 1, 2015. DOI: 10.1515/cdbme-2015-0110 (cit. on p. 48).

[61] R. L. Lieber, B. M. Fazeli, and M. J. Botte, "Architecture of selected wrist flexor and extensor muscles", *The Journal of Hand Surgery*, vol. 15, no. 2, pp. 244–250, 1990. DOI: 10.1016/0363-5023(90)90103-x (cit. on p. 49).

[62] R. L. Lieber, M. D. Jacobson, B. M. Fazeli, R. A. Abrams, and M. J. Botte, "Architecture of selected muscles of the arm and forearm: Anatomy and implications for tendon transfer", *The Journal of Hand Surgery*, vol. 17, no. 5, pp. 787–798, 1992. DOI: 10.1016/0363-5023(92)90444-t (cit. on p. 49).

[63] M. D. E.-D. Safwat and E. M. Abdel-Meguid, "Distribution of terminal nerve entry points to the flexor and extensor groups of forearm muscles: An anatomical study.", *Folia morphologica*, vol. 66, pp. 83–93, 2007, ISSN: 0015-5659 (cit. on p. 49).

[64] N. Malesevic, L. Popovic, G. Bijelic, and G. Kvascev, "Muscle twitch responses for shaping the multi-pad electrode for functional electrical stimulation", *Journal of Automatic Control*, vol. 20, no. 1, pp. 53–58, 2010. DOI: 10.2298/jac1001053m (cit. on pp. 53, 81).

[65] N. M. Malešević, L. Z. Popović, L. Schwirtlich, and D. B. Popović, "Distributed low-frequency functional electrical stimulation delays muscle fatigue compared to conventional stimulation", *Muscle & Nerve*, vol. 42, no. 4, pp. 556–562, 2010. DOI: 10.1002/mus.21736 (cit. on pp. 55, 56, 81).

[66] R. Nguyen, K. Masani, S. Micera, M. Morari, and M. R. Popovic, "Spatially distributed sequential stimulation reduces fatigue in paralyzed triceps surae muscles: A case study", *Artificial Organs*, vol. 35, no. 12, pp. 1174–1180, 2011. DOI: 10.1111/j.1525-1594.2010.01195.x (cit. on pp. 55, 56).

[67] D. G. Sayenko, R. Nguyen, M. R. Popovic, and K. Masani, "Reducing muscle fatigue during transcutaneous neuromuscular electrical stimulation by spatially and sequentially distributing electrical stimulation sources", *European Journal of Applied Physiology*, vol. 114, no. 4, pp. 793–804, 2014. DOI: 10.1007/s00421-013-2807-4 (cit. on pp. 55, 56).

[68] D. G. Sayenko, R. Nguyen, T. Hirabayashi, M. R. Popovic, and K. Masani, "Method to reduce muscle fatigue during transcutaneous neuromuscular electrical stimulation in major knee and ankle muscle groups", *Neurorehabilitation and Neural Repair*, vol. 29, no. 8, pp. 722–733, 2015. DOI: 10.1177/1545968314565463 (cit. on pp. 55, 56).

[69] L. Z. P. Maneski, N. M. Malešević, A. M. Savić, T. Keller, and D. B. Popović, "Surface-distributed low-frequency asynchronous stimulation delays fatigue of stimulated muscles", *Muscle & Nerve*, vol. 48, no. 6, pp. 930–937, 2013. DOI: 10.1002/mus.23840 (cit. on pp. 55, 56, 81).

[70] A. D. Koutsou, J. C. Moreno, A. J. del Ama, E. Rocon, and J. L. Pons, "Advances in selective activation of muscles for non-invasive motor neuroprostheses", *Journal of NeuroEngineering and Rehabilitation*, vol. 13, no. 1, 2016. DOI: 10.1186/s12984-016-0165-2 (cit. on pp. 58, 81).

[71] M. Krenn, U. S. Hofstoetter, S. M. Danner, K. Minassian, and W. Mayr, "Multielectrode array for transcutaneous lumbar posterior root stimulation", *Artificial Organs*, vol. 39, no. 10, pp. 834–840, 2015. DOI: 10.1111/aor.12616 (cit. on pp. 58, 60, 64).

[72] L. P. Kenney, B. W. Heller, A. T. Barker, M. L. Reeves, J. Healey, T. R. Good, G. Cooper, N. Sha, S. Prenton, A. Liu, and D. Howard, "A review of the design and clinical evaluation of the ShefStim array-based functional electrical stimulation system", *Medical Engineering & Physics*, vol. 38, no. 11, pp. 1159–1165, 2016. DOI: 10.1016/j.medengphy.2016.08.005 (cit. on pp. 58, 81, 83).

[73] S.-C. Chen, C.-H. Yu, C.-L. Liu, C.-H. Kuo, and S.-T. Hsu, "Design of surface electrode array applied for hand functional electrical stimulation in the variation of forearm gesture", in *12th Annual Conference of the International FES Society November 2007 – Philadelphia, PA USA*, 2007 (cit. on p. 58).

[74] Axelgaard Manufacturing Co., Ltd., *AG730 Stimulating Gel*, URL: https://www.axelgaard.com/Docs/TDS_AG730.pdf, Accessed: 13 April 2018 (cit. on p. 58).

[75] M.-S. Poboroniuc, D.-C. Irimia, A. Curteza, V. Cretu, and L. Macovei, "Improved neuroprostheses by means of knitted textiles electrodes used for functional electrical stimulation", in *2016 International Conference and Exposition on Electrical and Power Engineering (EPE)*, Institute of Electrical and Electronics Engineers (IEEE), 2016. DOI: 10.1109/icepe.2016.7781355 (cit. on p. 58).

[76] R. McLaren, F. Joseph, C. Baguley, and D. Taylor, "A review of e-textiles in neurological rehabilitation: How close are we?", *Journal of NeuroEngineering and Rehabilitation*, vol. 13, no. 1, 2016. DOI: 10.1186/s12984-016-0167-0 (cit. on p. 58).

[77] K. Yang, C. Freeman, R. Torah, S. Beeby, and J. Tudor, "Screen printed fabric electrode array for wearable functional electrical stimulation", *Sensors and Actuators A: Physical*, vol. 213, pp. 108–115, 2014. DOI: 10.1016/j.sna.2014.03.025 (cit. on p. 58).

[78] H. Zhou, Y. Lu, W. Chen, Z. Wu, H. Zou, L. Krundel, and G. Li, "Stimulating the comfort of textile electrodes in wearable neuromuscular electrical stimulation", *Sensors*, vol. 15, no. 7, pp. 17 241–17 257, 2015. DOI: 10.3390/s150717241 (cit. on p. 58).

[79] J. C. Batchelor and A. J. Casson, "Inkjet printed ECG electrodes for long term biosignal monitoring in personalized and ubiquitous healthcare", in *2015 37th Annual International Conference of the IEEE Engineering in Medicine and Biology Society (EMBC)*, Institute of Electrical and Electronics Engineers (IEEE), 2015. DOI: 10.1109/embc.2015.7319274 (cit. on p. 60).

[80] O. Schill, R. Rupp, C. Pylatiuk, S. Schulz, and M. Reischl, "Automatic adaptation of a self-adhesive multi-electrode array for active wrist joint stabilization in tetraplegic SCI individuals", in *2009 IEEE Toronto International Conference Science and Technology for Humanity (TIC-STH)*, Institute of Electrical and Electronics Engineers (IEEE), 2009. DOI: 10.1109/tic-sth.2009.5444408 (cit. on pp. 63, 64, 69).

[81] T. Exell, C. Freeman, K. Meadmore, A.-M. Hughes, E. Hallewell, and J. Burridge, "Optimisation of hand posture stimulation using an electrode array and iterative learning control", *Journal of Automatic Control*, vol. 21, no. 1, pp. 1–5, 2013. DOI: 10.2298/jac1301001e (cit. on pp. 64, 69, 81, 83).

[82] J. C. Loitz, A. Reinert, A.-K. Neumann, F. Quandt, D. Schroeder, and W. H. Krautschneider, "A flexible standalone system with integrated sensor feedback for multi-pad electrode FES of the hand", *Current Directions in Biomedical Engineering*, vol. 2, no. 1, 2016. DOI: 10.1515/cdbme-2016-0087 (cit. on p. 67).

[83] Atmel, *ATSAM3X8E*, URL: www.atmel.com/devices/atsam3x8e.aspx, Accessed: 13 April 2018 (cit. on pp. 68, 90).

[84] Arduino, *Arduino Due*, URL: https://www.arduino.cc/en/Main/arduinoBoardDue, Accessed: 13 April 2018 (cit. on p. 68).

[85] Maxim Integrated, *MAX7301 4-Wire-Interfaced, 2.5V to 5.5V, 20-Port and 28-Port I/O Expander*, URL: https://www.maximintegrated.com/en/products/interface/controllers-expanders/MAX7301.html, Accessed: 13 April 2018 (cit. on p. 68).

[86] Atmel, *ATmega328*, URL: http://www.atmel.com/devices/atmega328.aspx, Accessed: 13 April 2018 (cit. on p. 75).

[87] Texas Instruments Incorporated, *CC2540 SimpleLink Bluetooth low energy wireless MCU with USB*, URL: http://www.ti.com/product/CC2540, Accessed: 13 April 2018 (cit. on p. 75).

[88] DFRobot, *Bluno Nano - An Arduino Nano with Bluetooth 4.0*, URL: https://www.dfrobot.com/product-1122.html, Accessed: 13 April 2018 (cit. on p. 75).

[89] Maxim Integrated, *MAX6957 4-Wire-Interfaced, 2.5V to 5.5V, 20-Port and 28-Port LED Display Driver and I/O Expander*, URL: https://www.maximintegrated.com/en/products/power/display-power-control/MAX6957.html, Accessed: 13 April 2018 (cit. on p. 76).

[90] OMRON Corporation, *G3VM-351G MOS FET Relays*, URL: https://www.omron.com/ecb/products/pdf/en-g3vm_351g.pdf, Accessed: 13 April 2018 (cit. on p. 76).

[91] M. Lawrence, A. Brunschweiler, and T. Keller, "Multi-channel transcutaneous electrical stimulation environment.", in *International Functional Electrical Stimulation Society Conference*, Zao, Japan, 2006, pp. 210–212 (cit. on pp. 81, 83).

[92] J. Malešević, M. Štrbac, M. Isaković, V. Kojić, L. Konstantinović, A. Vidaković, S. Dedijer, M. Kostić, and T. Keller, "Evolution of surface motor activation zones in hemiplegic patients during 20 sessions of FES therapy with multi-pad electrodes", *European Journal of Translational Myology*, vol. 26, no. 2, 2016. DOI: 10.4081/ejtm.2016.6059 (cit. on pp. 81–83).

[93] M. Valtin, T. Schauer, C. Behling, M. Daniel, and M. Weber, "COMBINED STIMULATION AND MEASUREMENT SYSTEM FOR ARRAY ELECTRODES", in *Proceedings of the International Conference on Biomedical Electronics and Devices*, Scitepress, 2012. DOI: 10.5220/0003786303450349 (cit. on pp. 81, 83).

[94] M. Valtin, K. Kociemba, C. Behling, B. Kuberski, S. Becker, and T. Schauer, "RehaMovePro: A versatile mobile stimulation system for transcutaneous FES applications", *European Journal of Translational Myology*, vol. 26, no. 3, 2016. DOI: 10.4081/ejtm.2016.6076 (cit. on pp. 81–83).

[95] T. Keller, M. R. Popovic, I. P. Pappas, and P.-Y. Müller, "Transcutaneous functional electrical stimulator 'compex motion'.", *Artificial organs*, vol. 26, pp. 219–223, 2002, ISSN: 0160-564X (cit. on p. 83).

[96] A. I. Kottink, L. J. Oostendorp, J. H. Buurke, A. V. Nene, H. J. Hermens, and M. J. IJzerman, "The orthotic effect of functional electrical stimulation on the improvement of walking in stroke patients with a dropped foot: A systematic review", *Artificial Organs*, vol. 28, no. 6, pp. 577–586, 2004. DOI: 10.1111/j. 1525-1594.2004.07310.x (cit. on p. 86).

[97] R. Rupp and H. J. Gerner, "Neuroprosthetics of the upper extremity — clinical application in spinal cord injury and challenges for the future", in *Operative Neuromodulation*, Springer Nature, 2007, pp. 419–426. DOI: 10.1007/978-3-211-33079-1_55 (cit. on pp. 86, 89).

[98] J. Cauraugh, K. Light, S. Kim, M. Thigpen, and A. Behrman, "Chronic motor dysfunction after stroke : Recovering wrist and finger extension by electromyography-triggered neuromuscular stimulation", *Stroke*, vol. 31, no. 6, pp. 1360–1364, 2000. DOI: 10.1161/01.str.31.6.1360 (cit. on p. 86).

[99] J. H. Cauraugh and S. Kim, "Two coupled motor recovery protocols are better than one: Electromyogram-triggered neuromuscular stimulation and bilateral movements", *Stroke*, vol. 33, no. 6, pp. 1589–1594, 2002. DOI: 10.1161/01. str.0000016926.77114.a6 (cit. on p. 86).

[100] MED-El, *STIWELL med4*, URL: https://stiwell.medel.com/en/home? skipredirection=true, Accessed: 13 April 2018 (cit. on p. 86).

[101] TQ-Systems, *Mentastim*, URL: https://www.mentastim.com/startseite-mentastim (cit. on p. 86).

[102] J. R. Wolpaw, N. Birbaumer, D. J. McFarland, G. Pfurtscheller, and T. M. Vaughan, "Brain–computer interfaces for communication and control", *Clinical Neurophysiology*, vol. 113, no. 6, pp. 767–791, 2002. DOI: 10.1016/s1388-2457(02)00057-3 (cit. on p. 87).

[103] C. E. Bouton, A. Shaikhouni, N. V. Annetta, M. A. Bockbrader, D. A. Friedenberg, D. M. Nielson, G. Sharma, P. B. Sederberg, B. C. Glenn, W. J. Mysiw, A. G. Morgan, M. Deogaonkar, and A. R. Rezai, "Restoring cortical control of functional movement in a human with quadriplegia", *Nature*, vol. 533, no. 7602, pp. 247–250, 2016. DOI: 10.1038/nature17435 (cit. on p. 87).

[104] Texas Instruments Incorporated, *ADS1299 Low-Noise, 8-Channel, 24-Bit Analog-to-Digital Converter for Biopotential Measurements*, URL: http://www. ti.com/product/ADS1299, Accessed: 13 April 2018 (cit. on p. 90).

[105] A. Reinert, J. C. Loitz, F. Quandt, D. Schroeder, and W. H. Krautschneider, "Smart control for functional electrical stimulation with optimal pulse intensity", *Current Directions in Biomedical Engineering*, vol. 2, no. 1, 2016. DOI: 10.1515/cdbme-2016-0088 (cit. on p. 92).

[106] B. Dreibati, C. Lavet, A. Pinti, and G. Poumarat, "Influence of electrical stimulation frequency on skeletal muscle force and fatigue", *Annals of Physical and Rehabilitation Medicine*, vol. 53, no. 4, pp. 266–277, 2010. DOI: 10.1016/j. rehab.2010.03.004 (cit. on p. 103).

[107] M. B. Kebaetse, S. C. Lee, T. E. Johnston, and S. A. Binder-Macleod, "Strategies that improve paralyzed human quadriceps femoris muscle performance during repetitive, nonisometric contractions", *Archives of Physical Medicine and Rehabilitation*, vol. 86, no. 11, pp. 2157–2164, 2005. DOI: 10.1016/j.apmr. 2005.06.011 (cit. on p. 103).

[108] K. H. Gerrits, M. J. Beltman, P. A. Koppe, H. Konijnenbelt, P. D. Elich, A. de Haan, and T. W. Janssen, "Isometric muscle function of knee extensors and the relation with functional performance in patients with stroke", *Archives of Physical Medicine and Rehabilitation*, vol. 90, no. 3, pp. 480–487, 2009. DOI: 10.1016/j.apmr.2008.09.562 (cit. on p. 103).

[109] F. Quandt, J. Feldheim, J. Loitz, D. Wolff, M. Rohm, R. Rupp, W. Krautschneider, and F. Hummel, "EP 5. decrement of the effect of neuromuscular electrical stimulation over time in chronic stroke patients", *Clinical Neurophysiology*, vol. 127, no. 9, e234–e235, 2016. DOI: 10.1016/j.clinph.2016.05.061 (cit. on p. 103).

[110] H. Rouhani, K. E. Rodriguez, A. J. Bergquist, K. Masani, and M. R. Popovic, "Minimizing muscle fatigue through optimization of electrical stimulation parameters", *Journal of Biomedical Engineering and Informatics*, vol. 3, no. 1, 2017. DOI: 10.5430/jbei.v3n1p33 (cit. on p. 110).

Appendix A

Smartphone Controlled Electrical Stimulation

This section shall present a short guide of how to control the MOTIONSTIM 8 with an android device. The first step is to enter the ScienceMode on the MOTIONSTIM 8. Please refer to the MOTIONSTIM 8 user manual for instructions of how to enter the ScienceMode. In the second step the Smartstim adapter has to be connected to the MOTIONSTIM 8 (to the Mini-DIN 7 and RJ45 jack). If array electrodes shall be used Switchbox II has to be connected to the Smartstim adapter as well with a 6 wire flat ribbon cable. The output from stimulation channel 1 of the MOTIONSTIM 8 has to be connected to the two female jacks next to the 6 pin connector. One or two array electrodes can be connected to Switchbox II. One or two indifferent electrodes can be connected to Switchbox II by using the according connections next to the 16 pin connectors. The set-up can be seen in Figure A.1 (taken by Nils Remer).

The Android application called *Test-App 04 Tabs* has to be installed on the Android device. Once the Android device has paired to the Smartstim adapter (connect to Bluno) electrodes on the array (if an array is used) and stimulation parameters can be set to perform wireless controlled stimulations (Figure A.2 and A.3).

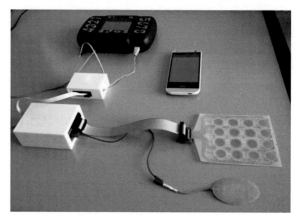

Fig. A.1. Set-up for wireless control with MOTIONSTIM 8, Smartstim adapter, Switchbox II and an inkjet printed array electrode.

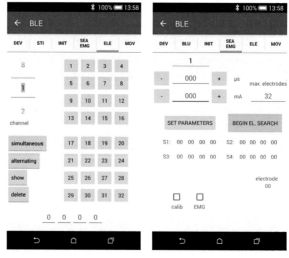

Fig. A.2. Electrode selection can be performed manually (left) or with the support of an electrode search function using flex sensors (right).

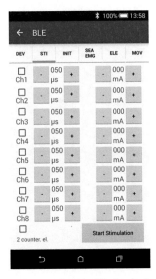

Fig. A.3. Stimulation parameters can be set with the Android application for each stimulation channel independently.

Appendix B

Fabrication of Array Electrodes

This section shall present a short guide of how to fabricate injekt printed array electrodes. To fabricate array electrodes an inkjet printer filled with printable silver ink is necessary. Such a set-up exists at the point of writing at the Institute of Nano- and Medical Electronics at the Hamburg University of Technology. A high resolution image or a vector graphic of the desired electrode layout has to be generated (Figure B.1 left). The electrode layout can then be printed on an adequate polyester film (in this project polyester films provided by the manufacturer of the silver ink were used). The next step is to fabricate an insulation layer. Therefore, a layout of the insulation layer has to be generated and printed on an polyester film with an adhesive side. The contact for the single electrode pads have to be punched out. In this project this was done manually with a hollow puncher. It is also required to leave out conductive material to connect a wire to the array electrode. An flexible flat cable (FFC) connector can be used for that purpose. It might be necessary to reinforce the the part of the array electrode used as the contact for the FFC connector to ensure a stable contact. Once the insulation layer is attached to the conductive layer the electrode is nearly complete. A conductive Hydrogel layer or liquid hydrogel shall be used to achieve a good skin contact. Dependent on the adhesiveness of the used hydrogel a bandage or a sleeve might be needed to attache the array electrode tightly to the body of the subject.

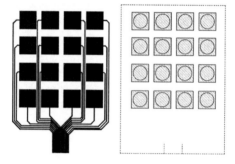

Fig. B.1. Ink-jet printed array electrode components. Substrate film with conductive
pattern (left) and insulation layer with marks to punch out electrode
contacts right). The marks for the electrode contacts are chosen in a
different shape and size compared to the conductive pattern to account for
inaccuracy during fabrication.

Lebenslauf

Name	Loitz
Vorname	Jan Claudio
Staatsangehörigkeit	deutsch
Geburtsdatum	19.07.1987
Geburtsort, -land	Bad Oldesloe, Deutschland

06.1994 - 06.1998	Grundschule Hoisbüttel
08.1998 - 06.2007	Gymnasium Ohlstedt
10.2007 - 04.2011	Studium Allgemeine Ingenieurwissenschaften
	Technische Universität Hamburg-Harburg
	Abschluss: Bachelor of Science
04.2011 - 11.2013	Studium Mediziningenieurwesen
	Technische Universität Hamburg-Harburg
	Abschluss: Master of Science
11.2013 - 04.2017	Wissenschaftlicher Mitarbeiter
	Institute für Nano- und Medizinelektronik, TUHH, Hamburg
	Projekt : ESiMED
04.2017 - Heute	Wissenschaftlich-Technische Leitung
	MEDEL Medizinische Elektronik
	Handelsgesellschaft mbH, Hamburg

Bisher erschienene Bände der Reihe

Wissenschaftliche Beiträge zur Medizinelektronik

ISSN 2190-3905

Alle erschienenen Bücher können unter der angegebenen ISBN-Nummer direkt online
(http://www.logos-verlag.de) oder per Fax (030 - 42 85 10 92) beim Logos Verlag
Berlin bestellt werden.